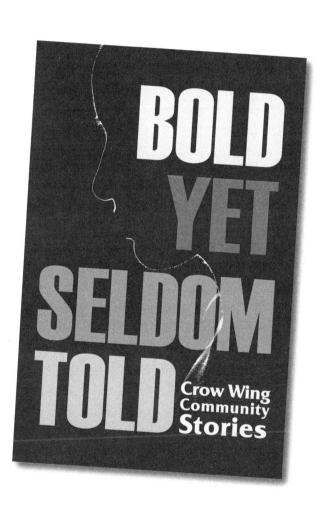

BOLD YET SELDOM TOLD
Crow Wing Community Stories

ISBN: 979-8-9891917-2-7

Design & Production: RiverPlace Communication Arts
  riverplacepress.com
  chip@riverplace-mn.com

Krista Soukup, Blue Cottage Agency
  Bluecottageagency.com

To order additional copies of this book, go to: https://crowwingenergized.org and send us a message on the contact tab.

Some of the authors recorded their stories. The videos can be found on https://crowwingenergized.org website.

This activity is made possible by the voters of Minnesota through a grant from the Five Wings Arts Council, thanks to a legislative appropriation from the Arts and Cultural Heritage Fund.

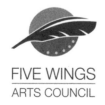

FIVE WINGS
ARTS COUNCIL

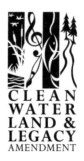

CLEAN
WATER
LAND &
LEGACY
AMENDMENT

Table of Contents

Table of Contents

Introduction

This volume of stories, poems and art was conceived during the beginning of the Covid 19 pandemic. Karen Johnson and I attended a virtual workshop organized by the MN Department of Health and Family Wise Services titled "100 Cups of Coffee." The research design was by Melissa Adolphson of Wilder Research and was based on the idea that too often people who make policies and design programs are out of touch with the people they are supposed to serve. We decided to change the name of the project to "100 Community Conversations," trained 10 volunteer interviewers, and began interviewing marginalized people with a connection to Crow Wing County.

The broad criteria for interviewing people were those who are closest to the problems but furthest removed from organizational decision making. We operationally defined that as those people with lived experience of mental illness, addiction, disability, incarceration, black or brown skins and LGBTQ+ folks. In some cases we interviewed the parents, grandparents, or caretakers of these people.

Among the interviewers, we had an experience of "empathy stretch." To sit down with someone with life experiences different from our own gave us insight into and compassion for people who are often stereotyped and seen as less than "normal" or "good" people. It was decided that we may be able to improve the mental and social-emotional health of our community by telling the stories of these marginalized people.

All contributors to this work have had a connection to Crow Wing County at some time. They may not presently reside in the county, but all have spent portions of their lives inside our geographic boundaries. Some of the experiences referred to did not actually happen in Crow Wing County, but none the less have affected the lives of the contributors.

Some portions of this volume may be hard to process for some readers, as the content can be raw and unfiltered at times. Try to remember that the authors are voicing their personal perspectives and memories, and that perception and memory are real for these contributors.

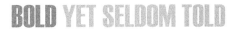

Bold Yet Seldom Told is our book and video series effort to create a more compassionate and belonging community. We hope your thinking and emotions are stimulated by these stories, poems and artwork. Please talk about your reactions with family, friends, and co-workers. Together we can create healthier connections and communities by honestly sharing what is same and different in our lives.

For those of you interested in digging deeper into the issues and meaning contained in the book's art and writings, please check out the Reader's Guide starting on page 107.

Lowell Johnson
Bold Yet Seldom Told Project Director

To order additional copies of this book, go to: **https://crowwingenergized.org** and send us a message on the contact tab.

Some of the authors recorded their stories. The videos can be found on **https://crowwingenergized.org** website.

Addiction Doesn't Discriminate...
But Neither Does Recovery

By DJ Osborne

My name is DJ and I am an addict. Always have been. I remember stealing whiskey at twelve years old. The first time I ever got drunk, my anxiety slipped away and I could do anything, thus beginning years of active addiction. I stole more alcohol and frequently drank alone. I got so depressed that I sliced my wrists often. At sixteen, I was diagnosed with GAD and MDD and I drank most of high school away.

At nineteen, I met my husband and childrens' dad. He was sober then, so I mostly stopped drinking, or at least didn't drink around him. Someone bought us wine for our wedding. We drank it together and were obliterated that whole week. Alcohol amplified poor mental health and caused a plethora of problems in our marriage, to the point of divorce.

Though I had been kicked out and physically carried out of bars, dripping in my own vomit, I went to the bar with a coworker one night. We paid our tab in quarters and ended the night at his buddy's house. My friend brought out a fistful of needles, a bag of rocks, and a spoon. He offered me some. It scared me, so I said no. His buddy chopped up a line of coke and I snorted it. That euphoria... I felt instantly sober, my depression and anxiety were gone, I had never experienced energy like that, and I felt powerful again. I was told that there was more meth if I wanted more. Confused, I scoffed, "I don't do meth." He replied, "Well you just did."

From then on, I remained drunk and loaded. I lost my job, our apartment, and eventually resided alone in my car. My boys were with their dad more often now but when I had them, I brought them to stay at my dad's with me. I had broken so many bridges and hurt everyone. He was about the only one who still seemed to care if I lived or died. I lied and stole and constantly bailed on those that counted on me.

My son had been fighting an infection under his jaw and his dentist abruptly sent us to Children's Hospital. This was my first day sober in many months... and not by choice. I tried to find drugs before we left town and even the whole couple hour drive to the hospital, but I couldn't. I was forced to go sober.

We were rushed through registration and they hooked my son up to an IV. They ran tests and a CT scan. Later that day, four doctors flooded our room to tell me that my four year old had cancer. I absolutely fell apart. My ex-husband arrived and we spent five days there. After many foxhole prayers and a succession of tests, our doctor concluded that it was a rare infection, curable with special antibiotics. I took this as a formidable warning from the Higher Power I only sought through necessity.

I found two places in town that offered recovery meetings and I showed up several times before psyching myself out and leaving. My spirit was broken. One night, I eventually pushed myself into that room full of people and my heart raced. I sat down next to a girl I had judged many years prior for her drug use. I melted. I was given hugs and thanked for being there. I kept coming back.

Right around that time, my boys and I moved in with my dad. We now had a safe place to live... together. I found a sponsor, worked the steps, and started making decisions conducive to the life I wanted. It took me nearly two years of relapsing and getting back up, but I was finally able to string some clean time together. I needed to find myself again so I started painting, something I hadn't done in many years. It was a way for me to release some of those heavy emotions I previously tried to drown in drugs.

I had eight months sober when a good friend and I were "voluntold" to start a meeting of our own. We were there every week and we stayed clean. After a year of sobriety, our relationship evolved. We rented a place together and created a safe, healthy home. He is good to me and treats my boys like they're his own. I'm so grateful. We bought a house together last year.

I've been blessed immensely in recovery. I have a knowledgeable therapist and I sponsor other women. I have meaningful relationships with people and my Higher Power. I've kept the same job for five years and have showcased my artwork in over a dozen shows, including two month-long exhibits. Best of all, I get to be a highly present mom and have the desire to stay sober. I never thought I'd make it into recovery but today, I have five and a half years clean.

A Journey with Depression

By Adam Rees

Coming from a family with a history of mental illness on both my father and mother's side, I grew up knowing the importance of mental health and the dangers it posed if left untreated. It can devastate lives like untreated cancer and heart disease. My mother, a psychiatrist, ensured that her children knew it was ok to talk about feelings.

I found myself dealing with depression for the first time shortly after college as I was struggling to understand my professional future. Ironically, I had a degree in psychology and was working at a psychiatric hospital but didn't feel safe talking about my depression with co-workers. With my mother's encouragement I sought help from a therapist, which resulted in a better understanding of this illness and provided a process to heal.

Years later the depression returned when my work became extremely stressful and life balance was lost. Starting with anxiety, my regular sleep was disrupted, which manifested itself in exhaustion and eventually situational depression. I remembered my mother's voice to seek help and knew it was the right time to reach out, in this case to my family physician for treatment.

Trust is crucial! When a colleague, friend or family member reaches out, they need reassurance that they will be listened to respectfully and confidentiality will be maintained. Authentic relationships are not built on human judgement.

Socrates' statement, "the unexamined life is not worth living" can be restated that an important element of a meaningful life necessitates that we understand ourselves. Authentic self-knowledge must include both our strengths and weaknesses.

For me, depression is a chronic illness. It never goes away but lurks in the shadows of life. It starts with feelings of anxiety that make restful sleep a challenge. This has become my early warning signal to go my primary care provider to proactively address the disrupted sleep and manage the anxiety.

I also learned, that when adopted, lifestyle changes can prevent or at least reduce the likelihood of a reoccurrence of depression. For example, focusing on better sleep habits and leaning on my faith through prayer and support from fellow believers has been extremely helpful. With time, life brings new learnings to improve coping habits. Recently my spouse helped me change my eating habits and I found less weight makes sleep easier.

Ben Franklin said, "an ounce of prevention is worth a pound of cure." I now believe life is not a solo sport. We need a community to live well. Smooth sailing is only true in fairy tales. From time-to-time life throws us all a curveball and our community can help us readjust our sails, especially during life's storms. A trusted relationship with a primary care provider is critical to head off the depression as it took some time to find the right medicine and dosage. My wife knows the signs and provides invaluable real time support. I have found pursuit of materialism increases my depressive tendencies while time spent with friends combined with nature lifts my spirits. As I look back over 60 years of life my insights into this illness and personal coping system took time to develop and came from frequent trial by error within a supportive network of friends and family. I'd be lying if I didn't admit to some close calls with hopelessness.

I hope my story reduces the stigma around mental illness and encourages people to get professional help sooner. Just like a patient with diabetes or heart disease who needs to manage their health with medication and lifestyle choices we each need to know the signs of mental illness to live our best life. It's time we remove the stigma and "Make It OK" to talk about our mental health.

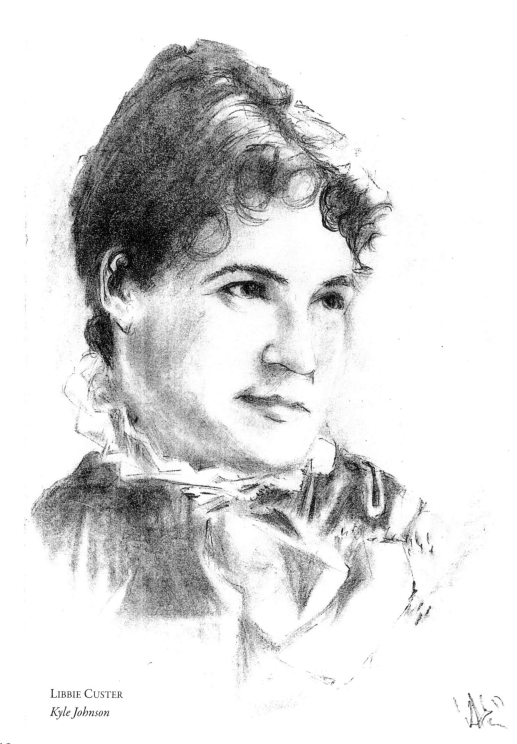

LIBBIE CUSTER
Kyle Johnson

Childhood Circles Known. And Not Known

By Patricia Adell Dickson

Shapes to color and try to draw
Playing fields for shooting marbles or scooping up jax
Birthstone rings and friendship bracelets
Counting how many . . . as the jump rope turned
Merry-go-round turning too fast or too slow
Going back home on the way to school: forgot the lunch
Ending an argument where it started
Neck scarves keeping winter cold at bay
Choreography for "A Tisket A Tasket"
A basket with green grass and colored eggs
Smoke rings Grandpa and my uncles blew
Soap bubbles dancing then bursting
Pathway for the ᵣrain under the Christmas tree
Wisemen, animals, shepherds around a manger
Twirling 8's with new skates at the park rink
Chasing front hall-through dining room-through kitchen-to front hall
Never aware that circles of rope were used to kill Black people

A Child A Community

"When a child is not embraced by her tribe, she will burn it down to feel its warmth." Ancient Proverb

By Ann C. Schwartz

Note: While the incidences in the following story could have happened anywhere in Minnesota, it is important to note that April attended school (K-12) in a different Minnesota county and later moved to Crow Wing County as an adult.

I could not understand why April seemed to sabotage what seemed to me to be every great opportunity, relationship, and potentially positive experience. She had everything. Her abilities, personality and passion for life were what I could only dream of having myself. She was fun, warm, smart, funny, athletic, passionate, and she was beautiful. I, on the other hand, was a head person who longed to be a heart person. I came from a stoic, achievement-oriented, competitive family riddled with dysfunction. I learned what it took to survive—be intelligent, responsible, successful in school and career, always be right, and always win. I admired and envied the person April was.

I always wanted kids; unfortunately, my husband and I could not have them biologically. I loved who I was when I was around children. It took no effort, at all, to operate from my heart. Around kids my guard dropped; I laughed, played, and loved. There was nothing I would not do to encourage, motivate, or protect a child. I didn't know it at the time, but I know now that I saw myself in them. It is what I needed from the adults around me when I was a kid but was lacking. I wanted to be the adult I wished I had had in my tribe.

My husband and I decided to adopt. We wanted to grow and learn more about the world, so we made the decision to adopt internationally. When we arrived in Bogota, Colombia to welcome our daughter into our family, our hearts melted and soared. We experienced her personality immediately. She was six weeks old, and full of love and expression. Her eyes were bright, and she had a smile that melted our hearts. Unfortunately, April had a deadly bacterium that the doctor could not eliminate. For weeks, between big, bright smiles, she would scream in pain. The doctors tried to gently prepare us by declaring that most adults would not live through it—the pain or the bacterium. April fought, and she survived. Doctors then promised us that she would be a force in this world. We had no doubt.

April is a healthy adult now. We couldn't be prouder of her. She is a wonderful mother of four beautiful children. She has embraced her community and has returned to college to pursue her passion to help others.

The doctors were right about April being a fighter, but what they didn't know was how much more difficult her life would be than that killer bacteria in her gut.

From a very young age, I could see that April would need to be strong and fight for herself. I witnessed how people saw her as less-than and how they felt that they had the right to get into her space and her face, because she was not like them, not white. When she was a toddler, touching her hair and body, adults would ask her where she got her soft, curly brown hair, her beautiful, striking brown eyes, her beautiful skin—because they could see that her parents looked very different. Their (maybe) well-intentioned compliments sent her the message that she didn't belong. When teachers had their students create a family tree and questioned hers, she got the message again. When, in her first year of high school, someone painted on her locker, "Go back to Cambodia, you N***** freak," she got the message again. And when April went to the office for help, she got the message loud and clear when she was instructed to go back to her locker where the janitor would bring her supplies so she could clean it off herself. The white girl did not receive so much as one hour in suspension. When that girl learned the power she had, she continued, relentlessly to bully April and others joined in. One day, when she pulled April down to the ground, from her backpack, April had enough and punched her. April got suspended, but the white girl avoided suspension again. When a police officer followed April's car, with two of her kids in it, for three miles and into our driveway and asked her what she was doing in this neighborhood, because she didn't look like she belonged here, she AND her kids got the message.

I taught April to stand up for herself. She watched me, and when I was tough and strong, and she saw me influencing the actions and thoughts of others, she took on the same approach. Only, when others said I was an articulate, smart leader with influence, she was told she was insubordinate, obstinate, and disrespectful. I got more unnecessary calls from school than any parent should have to address. I went to school, the office, the teachers, and I went to the school board to fight for her and all kids who were "different". No, April was not obstinate when she asked her teacher to explain the science lab in a different way so she could understand it. April was smart, and if the teacher had seen her differently than a brown student, he would've welcomed the opportunity to help all the class understand the two-page, single-spaced, typed instructions (without any illustrations) that I could not understand myself. When I went into the school office to explain the problem and insist that they let me into the science room to see for myself, they could not hide their utter amazement that I was April's mom; I was a white professional and destroyed their stereotypes. They let the white lady in. And when I used the instruments to explain and show April how to do the lab, she got it. Later that day in science, she helped other students in class who were afraid to speak up, by showing them how, and they got it too. The science teacher, embarrassed, requested that April be moved to another team because she was oppositional and defiant, and he didn't want her in his classroom.

When April reached her teens, we began to have trouble with the local police department. April was out past curfew, with her white friends. The police officer put April in the car and interrogated her, assuming she was up to no good. Granted, it was past curfew, but the other kids' parents were called and allowed to pick up their kids. We did not receive a call, until April had a melt-down, and the white officer wanted our help to calm her down. April told me that the officer had searched her purse, and found nothing, but took her camera. I met with the police chief and iterated my daughter's legal rights, along with my concern about the reason the officer took her into his car and interrogated her for an hour before calling us. I wanted to know what probable cause the officer had to take her camera, he left the room and returned with it without question. He apologized and agreed with me. He even gave his officer a warning—to stay away from April, for this was not the first time he had singled her out. I can't help but wonder if a brown mother would've received the same respect.

These include a very small sampling of April's struggles as she longed to feel belonging and acceptance for the beautiful human she is. What she learned at a young age was to not trust anyone, even herself. We never gave up hope, but she

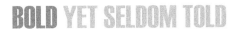

did, and she lost her faith in us, for we could not change the way people saw her. We felt helpless. April began to sabotage opportunities and experiences that promised to be different, better. She couldn't handle what she believed would be inevitable disappointment and heartache. She started skipping school; she faked illness to avoid social gatherings; she started using drugs to escape the pain. As parents, we were heartbroken and determined to raise awareness.

After years of hard work, April has found herself and her community. There were enough people who crossed her path along the way who saw her for the beautiful person she is, believed in her, encouraged her and helped her get back to who she was meant to be in this world. April believes in herself again, and she is a powerful force. She is using her experiences, insights, and strengths to help others. She accepts and lifts-up every human who is blessed enough to cross her path. She is a walking example of love and forgiveness, and no child who knows her will burn down any community that she is a part of because they know they are safe and loved in her presence.

Christine Grossman

As told to and transcribed by Pat Scott

Christine is a petite, blue-eyed blonde. She likes bright colors. She also has a quirky sense of humor and a hearty laugh.

Christine started life as the youngest of three children. She grew up in the Twin Cities and earned a bachelor's degree in 1985. Chris was married briefly. She recovered from a manic episode and got onto Social Security in 1997. "My [undergraduate] classmate in college … used to say that every month she had to have lunch with me to hear about the continuing adventures of Chris Grossman." Chris obtained a master's Degree in English in 1999. In 2001, she was starting a Ph.D. Program at UND Grand Forks, ND. She had to leave to care for her aging parents in Baxter. "It was a hard time."

After her father died in 2017, Chris was left with her Social Security and a small trust fund. She moved from one apartment to another. She was evicted from an apartment because her dog, a Cho weenie named Davy Jones, was bothering the other tenants.

In August of 2020, her difficulties snowballed. She didn't have money for her psychiatric medication. Her car ran out of gas on I94 and was impounded. She stayed in different homeless shelters in St. Cloud. "[When I was homeless and in the hospital with sepsis,] my brother died. His family is still mad at me because I didn't send my condolences."

"I was trying to stay at the YW [with her dog]. I saw this old woman outside having a cigarette. I told her I couldn't take him [Dave] where I was going…. Dave was at the elderly home with the elderly woman… I got shipped to Bismarck." When she returned to Brainerd, the County paid for a room at a budget motel. "[Living there] was bad! If you're there on County pay, even though continental breakfast is included for everybody else, the County pay people don't get anything." (Chris was apparently mistaken about this. She thought taking breakfast food was the reason she was evicted.)

BOLD YET SELDOM TOLD

On November 8, 2020, she was evicted from another motel without a penny to her name and taken to Prairie St. John's hospital in Fargo. The motel was supposed to be paid for by a delusional friend named David King. "I was in the hospital [Prairie St. John's] for my birthday. [The staff asked], why are you here? Most of these people don't even know they have a birthday."

Chris was committed to state care for six months. She was transferred to Rochester CBHH and later to the Wadena Specialty Hospital.

Chris said: "[It felt] Confusing, frustrating, humiliating. I kept trying to figure out how I had gone from a Ph.D. program to this situation. I mean, don't get me wrong, there are a lot of people with PhD's in English who have bipolar disorder. In fact, Catherine Zeta-Jones … and Jane Pauley both have bipolar disorder. So, I feel like I'm in pretty good company. …

"How did I get here? Why is this happening to me? What did I do to deserve this? And why aren't my parents still here so I could just be home?"

In March Chris was discharged from Wadena to an apartment in Remer. She retrieved her dog. However, on 8/28/21 she had to move again because of Dave's incessant barking when she was out. Again, she wound up in a series of homeless shelters in St. Cloud and later got a job working as a live-in personal care attendant for a man living in a dilapidated mobile home near Long Prairie. "I don't know how I survived all this. In the meantime, all my stuff was in storage."

She finally got into a ground floor 1-bedroom apartment at a new apartment complex for people with mental health challenges on 11/19/21 and has been there ever since. She did have to give up her dog. "It's a good apartment and there's a nice view. Sometimes they have bus tokens. The neighbors have problems…I'll just stay in my apartment with the door locked." After over a year of living there, Chris now has a personal care attendant (necessary because of worn-out knees and shoulders from 17 years as her parents' caregiver). She has finally been able to unpack boxes and decorate her apartment the way she likes it, including red area rugs. "It's nice to be settled for once. And the place is big enough to hold all my stuff." She belongs to a church and has friends she can talk to and cook for. Chris has recently joined the School District Community Education Board and has applied to a PhD program.

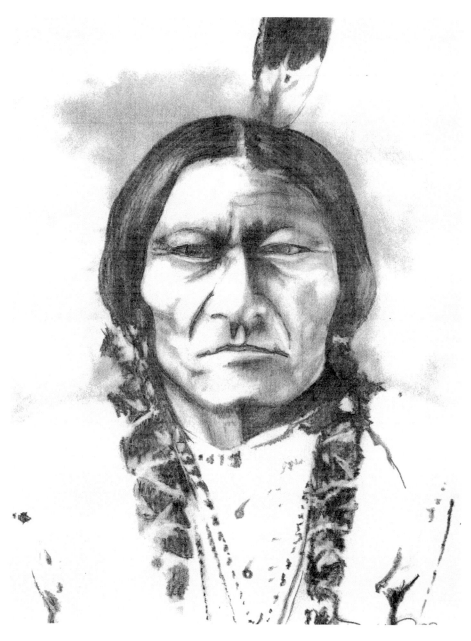

SITTING BULL
Damien Graham

Lost Souls

By Kayla Elwell

Depression is being a lost soul
He didn't want to let me go
He wanted me to be alone
Therefore, I wouldn't grow
I sat back and drank away
So, I wouldn't feel my pain
I'd cry
I'd scream, and more
Until depression would take hold
I didn't realize what was wrong
Before I knew it, me was gone
It wasn't me anymore
I realized I was a lost soul
I felt unworthy, weak, and betrayed
Then I realized this depression wasn't me
I have a voice so now I speak
I won't let depression take a hold of me
He had his time
He made me learn
He made me realize I'm not alone
Therefore, I'll stand tall
I'll walk and throw my bottles away
I'll take my time as I learn too
Take one day at a time!

One Family's Story

Anonymous

There are lessons to be learned when a family attends to the mental health needs of one of its members. But to recognize those lessons and embrace them is a whole other matter and none of it is easy. My family of origin is one of those families.

When I was younger, I always thought our family was pretty average and pretty normal. I felt safe and secure in the dynamics of my family. My parents had an intact relationship, older sibling who were successfully launched, no addiction issues, and no threats seemingly on the horizon.

I had just returned from two years in the Peace Corps, stationed in Africa. I had decided to go back to college to obtain my nursing degree, after spending those two years in Africa, working in part, with community/public health workers who I admired. I was living with my parents at the time when they received a telephone call from my brother-in-law, stating there was something wrong with my older sister. My sister and her husband were living on the east coast far from where I lived with my parents in Minnesota. My brother-in-law indicated my sister was acting strangely, and he could not get her to see a doctor or provider. He did not know what to do anymore and was fearful she would harm herself. He stated my sister was adamant she wanted a divorce. My father helped to arrange a flight back home to Minnesota and subsequently my sister was hospitalized for her mental health, although the time hospitalized was very brief. She was prescribed an anti-psychotic medication, determined not to be a threat to self or others and discharged to my parent's home.

Once home with my parents, my sister refused the medication prescribed. I was living at home during this time, and my parents, who were blue collar, high school graduates, were unable to comprehend fully what was happening to my sister. This was the 1980's before much was known about mental health crisis and resource availability. I, however, was in nursing school and had some idea what my sister was experiencing which appeared to be an almost catatonic state.

She barely ate or slept and would barely engage with anyone. My parents treated her gently. The first lesson learned. This condition was not her fault-and no amount of trying to demand she act differently was not going to help. They told my sister she could stay with them as long as needed to but they were concerned she would try and hurt herself. She told them she would not. This was also the reason she was discharged from the hospital, as she told providers she would not hurt herself, but there was every indication she was becoming a ghost to herself.

My sister started to take long solitary walks, and no one could find her. I took to looking for her as I was concerned, even if not suicidal, she would suddenly just disappear, get in a car and just leave. I found her one late afternoon-about a mile from our hometown walking along the river. Not only was I frustrated with the pace of her healing (remember she was still not taking medications and refusing to see another provider) but I started to resent her, because of the worry and distress and her continued refusal of care. I attempted to speak with her doctor from her hospitalization, stating we were so worried about her, but due to confidentiality he would not speak to me except to say until she is a risk to self or others there was nothing more he could do.

It was due to my increasing feelings of resentment and anger toward her that I learned the next lesson. You need a community. I joined the local NAMI (National Alliance of Mental Illness) and attended their support groups on a weekly basis. From these meetings, I found our family was not alone. I learned about mental health and brain function, trauma, and therapy. I learned, to give up on preconceived notions of what a healthy family and/or person looks like but to accept and help where you can in the present moment.

Ultimately with time and gentle care, my sister was one of the lucky ones. She became healthier with time, but it took a long time for her to fully recover. And yes, in time she used anti-depressants to help. Many months later, I spoke with my brother-in-law, and he stated prior to the change in my sister's mental health she had witnessed a significant trauma. Her co-worker shot himself in a completed suicide while at work. There were other aspects, which I believe, made this trauma hard for my sister to cope with including an emotionally distant partner, chronic cannabis use, and lack of social or family network.

If I could, I would wish for perfect health and happiness for everyone. But that is unrealistic, so instead I wish for letting go of the stigma of mental health and finding a community that is caring and supportive.

Erica's Story

Anonymous

Growing up in rural Minnesota has its' pros and cons. I grew up in the late 90's early 2000's when technology was beginning to emerge, but living 25 minutes out of town I was disconnected in a sense. We still only had access to dial up internet my graduating year of 2011. I had a fairly privileged childhood, until the recession hit around 2008. Both my parents were laid off from work and money was tight. My parents did the best they could and were able to bounce back.

I dealt with a lot of bullying and harassment in school. Being a neurodivergent kid without a diagnosis made it hard for me to socialize properly with my peers. Through middle school and into high school I became depressed and anxious. I began to self harm in 9th grade, my grades began to fall and I got into a fight with a fellow classmate from all the pain I was in. I did not feel supported in school by teachers and staff, mostly because mental health was still such a taboo thing to talk about. After the fight I, I was referred to LARJP to correct the harm that I had caused and to also remove the charge from my record. I made amends of my actions and believe that that experience put me back on track.

In the summer of 2012, my depression and anxiety came to a head and I decided to take my life. I attempted suicide by overdose of medication. I realized soon after I wrote my notes and taken the pills that I had made a mistake. I was rushed into the ER where the hospital staff was less than helpful in helping the mental state I was in. I spent 2 days in the ICU.

I feel like there is still a lot of progress that needs to be made in our community to be more inclusive, diverse and safe for all of our community members.

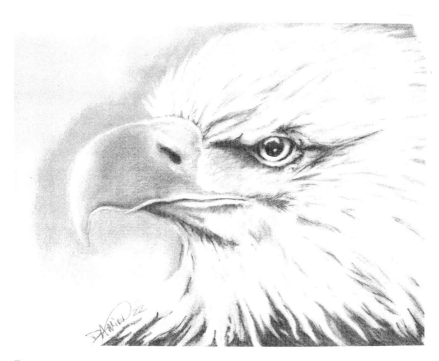

EAGLE
Damien Graham

The Aging Lesbian

By Joey Halverson

In this day and age, being an Aging Lesbian is just like being an Aging Anybody. So, I spoke to all the Aging Lesbians I have seen in the past two weeks to see what the overall thinking is.

We all discussed the difficulty of realizing you were a Lesbian in the '50s and '60s, how it was uncomfortable to share the loves of our lives with other people we cared about. Most people believed we were doomed to hell, and though they felt bad about that, they just wanted us to be "NORMAL". I even had a baby (not planned) to prove to myself I could be "NORMAL". It was at that point I knew God had made me exactly who I was meant to be and I did not have to be anyone other than my "NORMAL SELF".

This was 1970 and I was 27 years old. With that wonderful realization, I just became the best ME I could be. The more I accepted myself, the more others did also. I did not mind being OUT and OPEN when necessary, but I had no need to flaunt either. Just being ME felt so good I believe everybody around me felt good, too. (Tho I was a bit of a Pollyanna, so I suppose there were those who were still uncomfortable.)

I remember a day in the '80s when I was director of Community Action in Brainerd and someone made an aggressive remark about my "lifestyle" and questioned if that "is who we want to run Volunteer Activities in the Brainerd area"? Coming to my defense immediately was the local Sheriff, Frank Ball, who was also on my Board at Community Action. He told me, "Just keep being you, Joey, and know I always have your back." I believe I have been smiling ever since. This is the joy of living in a smaller community where people really care about each other, even if they have some doubts.

I have had a number of wonderful relationships with women, but none of them have lasted—as a "Lesbian Relationship". It could be that I usually chose women who were not Lesbians. They were friends I fell in love with. We would be together for a number of years and then they would realize this was just a break in their "NORMAL" routine and return to their usual lifestyle. The really marvelous part of this story is that they all remain my really good friends. I believe I can appreciate this aspect of my life because I had an awesome Astrologer who, back in the early '80s, told me that I was "destined" to live alone. That was hard to hear at the time, but now I know how really true it has become. I've lived alone for 20 years and never actually felt alone, as my friends have remained close and dear.

This reminds me of a workshop I attended in Minneapolis in the mid-70s when I was the Fitness Director at the Brainerd YMCA. We had to imagine our lives 5, 10 and 40 years from then. I saw myself in the 40-year future living in a small cabin in the northern desert lands of Arizona ....all alone ....with one dirt road leading to my hut. I was an artist and people would make their way to find me in the middle of nowhere. Right now, I live in Cinosam by myself, but in the middle of a caring and wonderful neighborhood, so I know I will not give that up to be in the desert......no matter how warm and comfortable that might be. I am where I am meant to be, for now.

As for Aging—I, and all the Lesbians I have been talking to, feel that being a Lesbian today is easier than Aging is. I want to thank all the people who have opened their minds and hearts to the Diversity of Life and have found the wonder in appreciating all of it. I have been a joyful recipient of all your Love.

Soliloquy #5

By Nathan David

Chasing my self around secret sounds, and lost
thoughts circling the once profound, shadowed.
And I follow by unhallowed ground.
He and I play hide-and-seek with darkness that
perpetually surrounds.

Definite in its campaign to see me riven and
below all with triumphant sadism that abounds,
Yet faith calls and disperses these follies without
an effort to be found.
Fatigued as the setting sun eclipses the moon,
beginning of more illusions cast by a tyrant of a
buffoon.

Tested and tried, my heart without divide,
I stand by the wayside, emotions colliding while
the will constantly dies.
And my smile cries without thoughts
torn from addictions and flaws, errant and
riddled through my life.

I dance with death yet refuse to die,
Myself troubled by myself and the voice that
constantly replies, mocked.
Yet death is toppled without the cornerstone
anywhere but hidden inside.
Seeking, but yet confused, this vortex of swirling
thoughts covex. (converge?)
I'm tired, yet before tyranny will I never relent.

Continued

Soliloquy: comes from the Latin *solus* "alone" and *loqui* "to speak." At its most basic level soliloquy refers to **the act of talking to oneself**, and more specifically describes the solo speech of an actor in a drama.

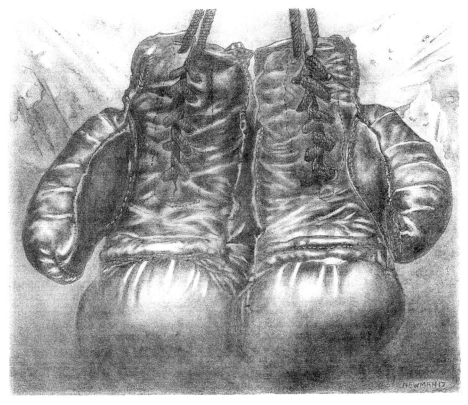

BOXING GLOVES
Ken Newman

29

Michael Samuel Abrego

By Michael Abrego

Hi. I'm Mike from Brainerd Minnesota. I had a long 25 year run in the dope game. Meth had such a grip on me.

I was a health nut, a good guy, a college graduate, and I had the world rooting for me until meth found me. The first time I tried meth was on a welding job in California. I had a bad hangover one morning from drinking after work at the hotel the night before. I didn't know it at the time, but some of the work crews were doing meth. I asked how they got up and got to work so early after drinking all night. I told a coworker I was too hungover and didn't feel like I would make it through the workday. That coworker said to meet him in one of the bathroom stalls and he would give me something to cure my hangover and make me feel better. He handed me a big line of what I thought was cocaine on his pocket notebook. At first I said, "I'm not doing cocaine—are you nuts?". It took some coaxing from him saying that it wasn't cocaine, but you do it like cocaine and to trust him and I'd be fine. So, I did my first line and it made me feel great, like I could do anything! I couldn't believe it. It really worked! I do, however, remember that I felt pretty shitty coming down from that yellow biker crank meth.

I knew it had to be bad for me, so I stopped before it got too bad. Unfortunately, in the next couple of years it started to show up everywhere. A newer and stronger form of crystal meth (or glass as we called it) made its way into my life. I remember thinking I shouldn't do any more, but I wanted to do more so bad. I got to a point where I said, "Fuck it, everyone else is doing it." I was hooked. I made my life revolve around it, and it didn't help that I gained big connections fast. I became a heavyweight supplier. I got hooked on being the plug for people. I actually made a lot of money, but I wasted it all and had nothing to show for it. I spent it all on more drugs, women, and gambling at casinos.

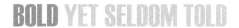

Suddenly, one day my main guy got busted. My life went downhill after nearly a decade of slinging meth, holding a job, and being a functioning addict. I wasn't able to get large quantities of dope to make any kind of decent profit. I started injecting myself, trying to numb out from my situation. At the same time I lost my welding job. I hung out with the wrong people. For the next 15 years I could only put a few months of clean time together. I lost two marriages, multiple jobs, and went through some bad tough spots losing family members to death. I went to treatment six times, two of which were outpatient. I've overdosed three times on heroin and meth and almost lost my life due to being robbed and getting in fights. I even went through the drug court program, but relapsed after two years.

The last time finally woke my ass up, as I nearly lost my life when I fell asleep at the wheel. I literally woke up in midair jumping my pickup at 70 mph over an approach, missing a telephone pole by an inch. I regained control after landing and pulled over on a side road to take a nap. I was so tired. I said a prayer to God to please help me as I couldn't quit on my own. I fell asleep and woke up to my prayers being answered by cops knocking on my window. I was so relieved and actually glad I was going to jail because I knew I could quit if I had help.

I went to treatment and then walked back into a Crystal Meth Anonymous (CMA) meeting that I had started 10 years prior when I was in Drug Court. Today I help chair the CMA meeting at the UpFront Alano Society in Brainerd. I have the best support system ever. On December 11, 2023, I will have been clean for three years! I have the world by the ass now. I have a great job, a great new family, and have my blood family's respect and love again, too. I have nice things, toys, and a nice roof over my head. It's all because of making a decision with God to quit. I think I was just so sick of my druggie life and ready to finally quit. I decided that I wanted to live and now I'm still here to watch my daughter and granddaughter grow through life with me as their happy-go-lucky grandpa and dad. I couldn't be happier.

The reason I've made it so far is this—I go to CMA meetings every Sunday, all year long. The three sayings that help me are: 1) If you always do what you always did, you will always get what you always got; 2) Nothing changes if nothing changes; and 3) Meeting makers make it. Because I am clean, I found the love of my life again. She is my high school sweetheart and after 30 plus years of being apart, we wound up back together. I think my higher power/God was waiting for me to get clean before He would allow me to have her. All those times I was using I was never in a healthy relationship. Now that I am finally clean and in a healthy relationship, my life is complete. She has actually helped me stay clean by going to all my meetings with me, even though she is not an addict herself. I am extremely grateful and lucky to have her in my life.

The CMA meetings we have at Up Front in Brainerd, Minnesota, make everyone feel like family. My sponsor, Jesse, is one of the best friends I've ever had. He's always there for me. We hang out and ride motorcycles, wheelers, and snowmobiles. Hobbies are so important.

In conclusion, having a God or higher power, a sponsor, working the 12 steps of CMA, having fun and healthy hobbies, consistently going to meetings every week, and having support is the best darn recipe for getting and staying clean. If I can do it, anyone can.

Thank you for reading my condensed story. I hope it helps someone in some way.

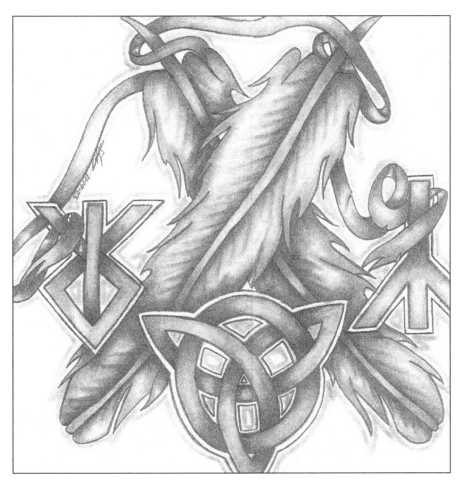

THE GOD'S PRAYER
Jessee Kuhns

Being Black in Rural Minnesota

By Donn C. Beaubien

Ever since college, in my places of employment I have been either the first, or only, Black female professional hired at the same level/position. While living in metropolitan areas, that reality in the work environment didn't seem to matter significantly, because in the larger community there were other Black professionals with whom I could connect. There also were Black theatre and Black organizations that offered opportunities for engagement.

My husband and I moved to the Brainerd Lakes area from the suburbs of the Twin Cities in 2007. When we bought our home in 2003, it was a place for us to retire. However, in the interim, I went to graduate school, earning a Master of Social Work degree and later becoming a Licensed Clinical Social Worker, specializing in grief therapy. When I was hired by Crow Wing County Social Services, I became its first (and to date, only) Black social worker. Later, when I transitioned to provide therapy at a mental health clinic, I remained without peers of any ethnic diversity for more than three years. My employment trend continued throughout my career.

Professionally, I was never personally insulted nor have I felt disrespected because of my race while working for the County in child protection or providing therapy at the clinic. Sometimes I wondered whether this was a reflection of my employer being the County, my age (60+ years at the time), or my profession as a mental health therapist. Therefore, for me, the primary challenge in living in rural Minnesota was not the professional environment but rather the scarcity of other minorities, and Black people in particular, with whom to identify and socialize. Secondly, the lack of Black cultural organizations has been a drawback.

As a *visible* minority I am more easily remembered. There are times when we all simply want to be alone—*invisible within a space*. But that is not possible when you are visually different. This visibility often creates some discomfort and uncertainty as well as limitations, such as causally browsing through small boutiques with a sense of being watched. In a metro area there would not be that type of discomfort.

Especially since the murder of George Floyd, many organizations have attempted to respond to social justice issues by addressing their commitment to diversity. Consequently, when I am invited to become a member of an organization or a board, the thought surfaces whether the ask is a means of checking-off the diversity box rather than seeking my skill-set. I doubt that thought would occur to most members of the majority. Similarly, there is often an underlying sense of being a representative for Black people. If I don't mesh well within an organization, will hiring/inviting the next Black person come with a degree of hesitancy? It is not uncommon for a Black person, or any minority, to feel the need to perform above average to pave the way for the next Black or minority professional.

Another challenge of being Black in rural Minnesota is the lack of seeing others like yourself within the glossy pages of promotional-type magazines. If there are no photos of Black people, how is the community encouraging diversity?

I mentioned earlier, I never have experienced any direct discriminatory interactions in the workplace. However, I have experienced discrimination in the greater community. Similar to many families in the Brainerd Lakes area, we are fortunate to live in a nice home on a lake. One day, responding to a knock at my door, a white man was inquiring about a house at a different address. I happened to know the residents about whom he was inquiring. However, he then asked, "do you live here?" Was he surprised that a Black person lives at this address? Would he have asked that question to a white woman if she had answered the door?

I have been asked where I am from because "you speak so well." And I recall, many years earlier, I was asked if I went to "elocution school." Most recently, I was asked why I came to the area. While the individuals who asked the questions seemed to mean well, as the receiver, I heard them differently—was there a stereotype of speech that I was not fitting into; is everyone asked why they moved here or is it because I am Black, and do I realize that there are not many here like me?

But for now, my husband and I continue to reside in the Brainerd Lakes area. And we continue to travel to the Twin Cities and elsewhere for the social, cultural and spiritual enrichment that feeds us.

Pain to Purpose

By Charly Rose Niesen

We all have a story, and over the years my story hasn't changed, but my view on it has and how I share it. As a teen I only knew dysfunction and chaos. I grew up in an addict / alcoholic and co-dependent home. By the time I was age 15 my father had been to 12 inpatient and outpatient treatment programs that I can remember. As you are reading this don't get me wrong. I do have many happy childhood memories but none in which my father was not under some mood-altering chemical.

Thankfully I was oblivious of his use as a child, but like many in addict homes I grew up faster than I should have. By age 15, my 16-year-old sister was already a mother and had her own struggles and we all lived under the same roof. Through the dysfunction and chaos, I was trying to find my place and role in my family, often feeling like I no longer fit since my niece had been born. She took the place that I once held as the youngest. So, to others what looked like me being rebellious was me needing attention. I started skipping school, drinking, stealing cars, and running away.

That definitely got me attention from my parents, teachers, and my peers and the Little Falls police department. I was removed from my home and put in many out of home placements from age 15 to 18 years of age. I was in CMRDC, Baxter youth shelter, St Croix girls boot camp, Grand Rapids foster home also Isanti ranch and several treatment centers. When I was in the many placements I would thrive and follow the rules and secretly loved the structure. I had my first child when I turned 18 years old, and at this point looking back I had never been modeled what a healthy relationship looked like. I settled for an unhealthy relationship that ended after less than a year as he was being unfaithful. At the time that I gave birth to my son, my own parents were going through a divorce so moving home wasn't an option. I soon settled into my own apartment with my newborn son, and still figuring out parenting. As a new mom and a young mom, I was sleep deprived and at times overwhelmed and lonely.

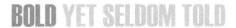

My son's father had seen him only a few times, and he would come at inconvenient times like 2:00 a.m. He would stay for an hour and leave, and this pattern continued for about a month. I finally said in person to him, "I am tired, and these late hours don't work for me. Why can't you come at normal hours?" He validated my feelings in one sentence and in the next said, "Charly, I have something to help you lose weight and have energy." This is the moment my life would change forever. I was introduced to methamphetamine.

He was right. I lost weight and had a burst of energy. I just wish he would have told me everything else I would lose. I soon lost my will to parent, my housing due to a domestic between us, and my self-respect and freedom. Once I found myself homeless, I asked my son's grandma to take him until I got back on my feet. I didn't expect that to take almost 7 years. My addiction had spiraled quickly. I went from snorting to smoking to intravenous use. I realize now that I just wanted to numb myself and not feel my pain.

After getting out of jail and being placed on probation I was able to get sober, and at one time I had 18 months clean. I was expecting my second child and was in a relationship at this point, the healthiest one that I had ever been in. Sadly, that explains a lot as it was mentally, physically, and verbally abusive. I found out I was expecting my second child, another boy, and at this time I was working at the workforce center and focusing on getting my GED. My boyfriend was also sober and had started a roofing job. We both had been preparing for the arrival of our son. July 31st, I gave birth to my second son, and my mom and my boyfriend's mom all supported us during delivery. We had settled in at home and baby was just shy of three weeks, when my Father called and wanted to come over to meet his new grandson as he had not met him yet.

When you hear people say addiction is powerful, cunning, and baffling, this is what they mean. I was sitting on the couch in the living room, had just finished nursing the baby, and my boyfriend had just left for work. My dad came in and brought his friend Brent who I also knew. He talked to me and admired his new grandson and within minutes said, "Charly, want to get high?"

At first, I was insulted by him asking but no sooner had I put the baby in his crib, than I came back to the living room and grabbed a mirror from my closet and snorted a line. I thought, if I don't IV use, I will be ok. That day everything, I had worked so hard for was lost within 24 hours. My boyfriend came home from work and relapsed that day. My dad left that evening and the next morning I received a knock at my door. It was my probation officer. She saw the state that

I was in and called the police and child protection. I went to jail, and I was served with papers for eviction and a child protection case. I went to treatment right from jail to Liberalis for a 120-day inpatient treatment program that I completed. I had a 16-month child protection case and met with 11 professionals on a weekly basis as part of my case plan. I would only get an hour visit a week with my children.

At times I felt defeated. With my past criminal history, I had many barriers when it came to employment and stable housing. Happily, this is the part of my story when things start to turn around. I was introduced to Kimberly Pilgrim and the program called Meta-5 MN family resiliency program. Meeting Kimberly for the first time, I was intimidated at first. She was a woman with confidence. She lit up the room. Kimberly didn't care what was on paper about me or my past; she allowed me to start believing I had a future. She taught me what integrity meant and believed in me when I wasn't able or ready to believe in myself. Kimberly created a safe place for many women, including me, who had child protection involvement past or present.

I don't want to speak about CPS, however. There is no easy child protection case. Even with Kimberly in my life, teaching me many life skills and being present at all my court hearings, it was very hard as I would sit and wait on the long, cold wooden benches outside of the courtroom. I was afraid of going into the courtroom, as I never knew what the outcome would be for that week.

Kimberly loved me to wellness, in a room full of professionals that I feared at the time. Amongst themselves, they would have a conversation. They spoke about me, but no one spoke to me. They spoke as if I wasn't present in that same room. Kimberly came into the room and slapped her hands on the round wooden table. Everyone jumped in that room, including me, as she said these words that forever changed my life. "You know what the problem is? Everyone forgot to tell Charly how magnificent she is." I had been called many things, but magnificent was not any of them. That day I sat up a little taller and thought maybe she is right. I knew she would never lie to me or about me.

During my time in Kimberly's program, I found out who my true authentic self was, and that I had a voice. I learned about what a healthy relationship was. I developed employment skills, and I received my GED. I was able to further my education through the program. I went from being homeless to now being a homeowner. I am married and have been with my husband for 18 years. We met when we both were struggling with addiction, but we created a life of recovery together. We have four children that we are raising together. I am a blessed mother of 7 beautiful children, ages 5 to 23 years of age.

When I became sober, I wanted my recovery to be louder than my addiction ever was. Currently working in the mental health field as a Certified Peer specialist and a recovery peer specialist, I have my certification as a Family peer specialist and a mental practitioner. I am also a WRAP facilitator. Wrap stands for wellness recovery action plan. I have been able to take my experience and help others from youth to adults. My current position is at FOCUS unit Essentia Health, the same chemical dependency treatment I found my recovery at a little over 17 years ago.

I am active in my community because the opposite of addiction is connection. I am part of (BLADE) Brainerd Lakes Area Drug Education, and (LARJP) Lakes Area Restorative Justice; am proudly a Meta-5 Mn Family resiliency alumnus; a national selling author in a book with 25 other women from all over the world; and am currently going to school fulltime, furthering my education to receive my AAS and Addiction study certificate to work as an LADC. I am not one to hold back so I dream BIG dreams and I am excited to see what the future holds. I want to travel, help social services redesign a few of the programs they currently have such as parent works. Hopefully one day I can start a family court in our Crow Wing area.

I have created a life I no longer need to run from. I no longer need to escape pain. It was never that I didn't love my older children. It was that I didn't love myself. I am proud to say I never used any chemicals during any of my pregnancies. And if you're wondering about my relationship with Kimberly, she is still in my life and my children's life, cheering me on, taking my calls when I want to share something positive, when I am ugly crying on the phone, when I need to process something or just thank her for always loving me. Therapy used to feel like a punishment, but as I have healed, and I am still healing parts of me, I realize what a privilege therapy is.

This is a story I share often: my old therapist asked me, "Charly, when will you know that you are successful?" To me it wasn't a job title, or a car. It had nothing to do with money. Instead it was having a Newton's cradle—the metal thing that has balls that you click together. So the first day I started at Essentia Health Focus Unit, that was the first thing that went on my desk. Every day that

I work, I click the Newton's cradle balls together to remind me this is what recovery and support and self-love have created. The things that you could have never dreamed of are now your reality. These are the promises you hear about in recovery. I have heard many quotes and sayings in recovery, and one that has never sat well with me is "Fake it till you make it."

You can say I "charlyfied" it: "Practice it until it becomes reality."

Butterfly Free

By Michael Corwin

Unlike the butterfly
I have no wings
I try to fly
But now I sing
I have one song
Not long to sit
Only one so strong
Alone in a pit
Hear my voice
I now will sing
Make a chance
To let freedom ring

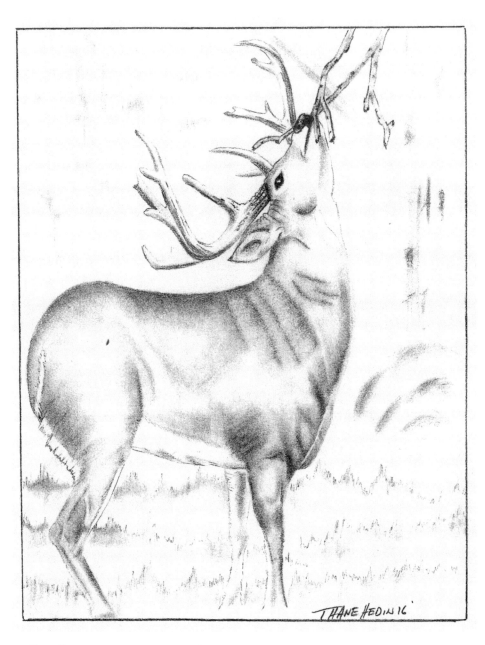

DEER SCRATCHES
Thane Hedin

Vicky

By Vicky Kinney

My son died of an accidental overdose a year ago. He was 31 years old, and I miss him every day. I wrote this for him for his funeral.

Jeffrey,
From the start I knew you would
      have challenges to face.
I couldn't pave the way for you
      as you searched to find your place.
There were days my heart would melt;
      you were so pure and kind.
You also marched to your own beat
      and I thought I'd lose my mind.
Your world was joy and turbulence,
      it's how you felt inside.
You couldn't break free from inner pain,
      no matter how you tried.
For years I failed as I tried to fix
      your life and burdened soul.
Then I learned to simply love you,
      knowing Christ would make you whole.
I'm grateful for all you brought me,
      aggravation, tears, and joy.
You became a man but with that grin,
      I still see my little boy.
You left this world and went on home.
      You had run your race.
You're free and whole and I'll hold you soon
      In the warmth of God's embrace.

Love, Mom

I Have Two Moms

By Prairie Smoke

I have two moms.

My birth mom "came out" when I was 21 years old, one year after my parents divorced after 20 years of marriage. I was the reason they married in the first place- Catholic cheerleader, made pregnant by the high school basketball player from the town over- they did what you did back then, they got married despite having known each other for only three months.

Sue, my other mom, came into our lives when I was in second grade. Mom met Sue at their job in a local factory—Sue a single woman at the start of her career, my mom a wife and mother of three girls, working the night shift to bring in some extra money. Their friendship grew slowly as they were both at different points in the journey of life. Yet Sue was one of her only friends and that friendship continued as we all grew older.

My sister Tracy and I were pretty sure Sue was gay, as over the 10+ years of their friendship, we had never seen Sue date a man, or really anyone for that matter. There were some late-night calls from Sue when she had too much to drink, with my mom whispering into the phone and then she and Dad arguing later. But there was NO WAY they could be more than friends—Mom was, after all, married to Dad—she had sex with him to create all three of us girls—she was Catholic—she thought Barry Manilow, Michael Bolton and the singer from White Snake were cute—no way was Mom gay.

My parent's marriage started to show serious signs of crumbling when I was in high school. Lots of fighting, crying, door slamming, driving off angry—my mom relying more and more on her bible and church. My dad started a 2nd job in the evenings at the bowling alley, spending less time at home to avoid arguing. When I was 20 years old, my parents divorced. Of course, it made me terribly sad- my family was no longer whole. But the adult side of me knew it was for the best. Neither of them had been happy for YEARS- heck, they only knew each other for 3 months before they decided to get married. Maybe they never really loved each other like they both deserved to be loved.

About a year after their divorce, (I at 21 years old, my sister Tracy at 16 years and sister Crystal at 12 years), Tracy and I, as well as our dad, starting hearing rumors around town of mom going to "gay parties". The image of a "gay party" in our naïve minds was one of wildness, nudity, unbridled freedoms that we KNEW our mom would never engage in. Tracy and I decided to approach my mom about it- to find out if what we were hearing was true- if it wasn't, of course we wanted to protect our mother from the rumors but if it was- there was further discussion to be had as there would be so many more questions.

That conversation with our mom resulted in her "coming out" right there in the kitchen with Tracy and I. "Yes, Sue and I are in a relationship." The "gay parties" were simply she and Sue hanging out at Sue's sister's house with her female partner. Just four lesbians, sipping cocktails, eating snacks, and playing board games on a Friday night- just like any group of friends may do. We learned she had been going to a support group in the metro to deal with her feelings, her Catholic values, and coming to terms with what this meant for her future. My sister Tracy was a bit upset, not quite old enough to grasp this response. I, being a bit older, felt okay about it. I was happy for my mom. Happy that she could finally say this to us and not have to hide her feelings about who she loved.

The rest of her coming out story didn't go quite as smoothly. When I first married at age 28, we wanted Sue to be a part of the day in the role she had assumed in our lives for the past 8 years now- Mom's partner. But Mom's Catholic, conservative-leaning family (11 brothers and sisters, 42 nieces and nephews, and a mom) didn't know about her relationship. Mom picked a sister and a brother that she thought would be supportive confide in first. Then she shared it with the others. Several of her siblings wouldn't come to my wedding, some stopped talking to her, others sent her Bible verses along with notes about the sins of her relationship, a few wouldn't go to the home she and Sue shared, while others blatantly ignored Sue at family gatherings.

With the support of me and my siblings, a handful of aunts and uncles, and most importantly GRANDMA, the road got less and less bumpy. Relationships have healed, although there are scars. And they endured. We endured. LOVE endured. I have such deep respect for Mom and Sue's relationship. They have now been together for over 27 years, marrying in 2015 when same sex marriage was legalized. They have a love like no other. They are a partnership. They are a team. There is no toxicity—only genuine respect and care for each other.

Having two moms is an amazing gift. I am glad I have two moms.

Micah's Story

By Micah Hudson

My name is Micah Hudson. I am 23 years old, and I was born mixed; half Caucasian and half African American. I want to share a unique experience of growing up as racial slurs don't mean much to me because of my split ethnicity; even when I found myself the target of racial discrimination and prejudice.

I believe what affected me the most growing up was everyone's else's confusion on what racial ethnicity I was. Because I was mixed, I often found myself in the "No-Man's Land" of racial identity. Whenever I meet a new group of individuals my ethnicity comes under question. The group tends to ask what my ethnicity is and tries to fit me into a cultural group. But because I am split this often leads to arguments about whether I am African American or Caucasian. When I was younger this often led to alienation among different groups. Whenever I found myself trying to hang with a group with a predominant ethnicity, such as a group predominately Black or Caucasian, they tend to bombard me with questions until they are satisfied in fitting me into whichever category they felt I fit in.

I was then expected to fit into that role and frequently they would make comments about how I did not fit the stereotype of that race. I believe because my ethnicity tends to be such a big deal when I join a social circle it becomes integrated in how they view me. These social groups tend to make comments about my music, my taste in movies, my favorite sports, etc. and make comments about how because I am black or white; it is weird that I didn't like this or that. Growing up I've always felt alienated; unable to feel a part of a particular culture. Every action of mine seemed to be under a magnifying glass ready to be vivisected. I often felt like I had to fill a role and found myself trying to fit these stereotypes to fit in. I even found myself submitting myself to constant racial jokes, reinforcing them to fit in even when I was constantly at the butt of the joke.

The sense of belonging and constant reminder that I did not belong was detrimental to my social health. Learning to communicate and interact in a social group fills me with an everlasting sense of anxiety and fear that I will say the wrong thing. My mixed racial identity puts me in the middle for every racial stereotype of the two races. I've been called and accused of every racial name, conspiracy, and prejudice comment possible. Early on in my youth it had a detrimental effect on my identity. I did not understand where I belonged and felt alienated, an outsider looking in.

Growing up it took some time to shrug these comments and stereotypes off, as well as realizing that I will never truly be accepted into a group. I will always be considered an outsider. It also took some time to learn how to communicate with strangers, which presents me with a certain amount of anxiety and dread. Now I get along much better than I used to. I volunteer and work with others so I can experience socializing with individuals and groups. However, I still feel the emotional trauma of not belonging will stick with me for as long as I live, no matter how hard I work to push through it.

My Journey

Anonymous

Are you gay? That was the question posed to me by a classmate in the 9th grade. Having grown up in a small conservative Lakes Area town in the 80's and early 90's; that was not a question I was willing to answer to myself or anyone else. The answer lied buried beneath denial and lies I told myself. Social pressure, both subtle and overt, taught me that the real me wasn't acceptable. Knowing you are not like others creates shame. Shame is the monster in your head that tells you are flawed. You feel that you are flawed at a very basic level and it must be covered up at all costs—as best as you can anyway. You are a sissy boy in a world that revers masculinity and it is NOT OK! That is the cross to bear for young gay men growing up in a heteronormative society.

I can remember being a young child and liking dolls more than trucks. That is how I first knew that I was "different". Parents know that their children have innate interests and personalities from a young age. These innate qualities are not chosen, they just are. It was just in my nature to gravitate more towards dolls. However, there was a clear discomfort from the men in my life. I can remember my mom helping me "smuggle" a new doll into the house past my dad. I don't blame my dad for this. Dads are not taught how to raise a son that is "different". Every new parent has a mental picture of what they envision theirs child's life will look like. When there is a departure from their template, it is hard for the parent to adjust their expectations for their child.

My love of dolls was the beginning of a long struggle to fit in and find acceptance. It was also my introduction to the feeling of shame. While many minority groups struggle to fit in, the unique thing about being gay is that you struggle to fit in with your own family. From the time you are very young, this basic need isn't being met. I had an idyllic childhood in so many ways. I had wonderful loving parents. I grew up on a lake. We seemed like the perfect middle class family. I had an older brother who was a star high school athlete and then there was me. I was the skinny blonde kid who got mistaken for a girl on occasion. I couldn't hit or throw a ball to save my life! I loved art. I would draw pictures of ladies in beautiful dresses. I knew these were feminine qualities. I was not proud of my gifts. Shame had reared its head.

Although I was a bit different, I had neighborhood friends. We would built forts or fish off the dock. I had girlfriends in elementary school. I even got married on the playground! Ha! Looking back, I was already romanticizing and modeling the heterosexual relationships I had observed. I already knew that I thought some boys were cute. Society tells you those feelings are wrong. Shame rears its head. It was the 1980's and AIDS was raging among gay men. In my mind, being gay meant a horrible death. I would have to bury those feeling to live a "normal" life. The template for my dysfunctional internal life had been set.

The insecurities that had taken shape would explode during my teen years. I grew taller and skinnier with the new addition of acne. Yay puberty! Ninth grade was like Lord of The Flies in Girbaud jeans. The social pecking order was ruthless. The alpha social girl group was out for blood. I had no friends at that point so I became the perfect victim. My love of name brand clothes did little to protect me from their venom. Shame rears its head. I just wanted to be invisible. I turned inward during those years. I was damaged in ways I didn't even realize. There were a few girls who were nice to me. I couldn't let myself get close to any of them though. "What kind of boy only has girls as friends?" I would ask myself. A gay boy, that's who! Shame had turned me into a loner. It was psychologically traumatic time for me. The emotional template that had begun to form during elementary school had been set. I felt like a circus freak in designer jeans. I walked the halls with my head hung low, steeling myself for someone to yell "fag" or have my books knocked out of my hands. I never thought of myself as a nerd though. I just felt misunderstood. I let very few people in well enough to get to know me.

After high school, I went onto college. Looking back, I know that I moved onto my college years still traumatized by my high school experience. I still didn't have much in common with most of the guys. I also still didn't want to be the guy with only girls as friends. I had boxed myself into an emotional prison. Even though I enjoyed my new freedom, I was still ostracized. There was the time I came home from class to see a derogatory gay term written on my dorm room white board. Another time I was walking behind a college jock. When he turned around he called me a fruit. Shame rears its head once again. I hated myself and I wanted to assimilate. Survival meant being like the others. I wanted to date and I wanted to date girls.

I convinced myself that I was bisexual. If I was bisexual, I could just turn off the part of me that I despised. I would then be able to survive in this world. There was a time when I felt like I might have to kill myself if my parents ever found out my secret. The gay equality revolution had not begun. Living a gay life in northern MN was not an option for me at that time.

In my junior year of college, I met the woman who would become my wife. We both went out with mutual friends one night. After that night, she began e-mailing me with interest. The fact that someone had taken a liking to me was intoxicating. She was like an angel who had been sent down to save me from myself. We began dating and it was great. I had a built in friend and it felt like I belonged somewhere. I was proud to be with her. I felt like I was living my dream. The dream of belonging and having the straight relationship I had romanticized. I loved her for loving me and saving me from myself.

It was Spring Semester of my senior year that we found out (surprise) that we were expecting. It was a scary and exciting time. I proposed to my girlfriend on the beach in Texas a couple weeks later. That time in my life was scary and uncertain but at least it gave me direction. I was going to be a dad and marry her mother. That settles that internal conflict!

My daughter was born in the fall of 1999. To say that I was unprepared for the responsibility of parenthood is an understatement. I needed work so I began working for my brother in the construction trades. Money was tight and our daughter had severe colic. I went from having very little responsibility to being a breadwinner. I was proud of my wife, daughter and picture perfect life. The fun of dating had given way to the pressures of parenting. My internal feelings were no longer being masked by fun and the adoration of my girlfriend. The disconnect between my authentic self and the life I was living had never been greater.

During the next years that followed, we would welcome two more children. I loved my family but I was struggling. When people think of someone in my situation, one thing comes to mind, the physical aspects of a romantic relationship. That was not the most difficult part for me. The hard part was trying to fit in once again. Heterosexual marriage is a construct of roles. Certain things are expected of women and certain things are expected of men. I was told more than once that husbands don't decorate. Ha! Once again shame was rearing its head in my life. I had to quiet the parts of myself that made me unique.

When heterosexual couples socialize together, husbands and wives tend to split up and have different conversations in different parts of the house. I always hated when women would leave the room. I was left having to rely on my limited knowledge of fishing, hunting and sports. Luckily I have a bit of knowledge from my dad dragging me along on his pursuits. Thank you, dad!

Once again, during this time I was without friends. I had a hard time relating to other husbands and fathers. I also distanced myself from female friends. When a "straight" married man has female friends, it raises questions. Is he interested in them romantically? Is he a closeted gay? My high school insecurities around not having friends and fitting in were back. The shame spiral was in full effect.

During my marriage I had two major emotional/mental breakdowns. Those were incredibly dark times. After the first episode, I was diagnosed with generalized anxiety disorder. I have struggle with anxiety since I was a child. I can remember several bouts of health related panic as a child. Every ailment was quickly diagnosed by my disordered brain as cancer. Yep...I was a fun kid! Ha!

All of the stresses, insecurities and shame culminated to a toxic level and lead to a complete system breakdown. I went days upon days without sleep. At my worst I would think of driving off the road and hitting a tree. During these periods medication saved me. I can remember the feeling of the "clouds" parting as the medication kicked in.

Eventually, my wife came to find out my truth. The details are personal but I will say that it did not involve cheating. She discovered my truth...that I was attracted to men. My poisonous truth was finally out in the open. Secrets are emotional poison. I had been sick with that poison for so long. It was terrifying and yet freeing that I didn't have to hide any longer. After some tearful conversations, we agreed to try to make our marriage work. For a time, one could even say that our bond was strengthened. She had a deeper understanding of me. Here was someone who knew my awful truth (as I saw it at the time) and still loved me. Over time, though, we became more like roommates. It changed her attraction to me. The secret had strengthened our friendship but killed her romantic feelings. She would go on to find someone who embodied the masculine traits that I lacked.

I don't feel like I went through the normal stages of divorce. I understood when my wife found another man. There was no rage. I didn't hate her. I was sad for our kids though. That was the hardest part. It still breaks my heart to think of the day we told them. They didn't know the exact reason behind the divorce for many months. The bright side was that I now got to live my truth. It was a time of guilt and sadness but also great excitement.

I lived with my parents for a time after my divorce. I had told them my truth the same night that I broke the news of my divorce They were completely supportive. After about six months, I moved into my own condo in Breezy Point. Once I was on my own, I tried to find a sense of community as a gay man in the Brainerd Lakes Area. I was hoping to find an active gay men's group in the area. A group with monthly meetings/events was what I was looking for. That does not exist here like it does in the Twin Cities.

I did a bit of dating once I was on my own. I was lucky to meet someone amazing straight out of the "gay gate". He is kind, compassionate and truly my soulmate. He could relate so well to my painful youth experiences. We had experienced the same hurts. We looked at life through the same lens. I am blessed to have found him.

My daughters accept us completely. It's been harder for my son. He has been affected by the conservative attitudes of the lakes area and society in general. He feels as if it is secret he needs to hide at all costs. There is shame in having a gay dad for him. He hasn't said that but it all boils down to shame. In turn, there is a new sense of shame for me. Shame changes form but it is always there for me. It's been an insidious feeling lurking around the every corner. It's there waiting to destroy whatever confidence or sense of peace I may have cultivated. My new life definitely hasn't been without bumps. My parents love and accept my partner and me. My brother's family is another story. Their Evangelical beliefs have prevented them from embracing my relationship. My brother has met my partner once. My partner has not met his wife and children. They do not want their children around THAT. We could get together with only them but not with the children. That is not acceptable to us. The idea the children need to be kept away from gay people is deeply offensive.

My flawed relationship with my brother reinforces all of the feelings of shame I have felt in my life I have had therapy to deal with the trauma of being rejected by a family member. When a family member makes you feel OTHER, it is a form of rejection. Family is the one place you are supposed to feel a sense of belonging. The opposite of belonging is rejection. When you don't validate my relationship, you are invalidating me as a person. I can't stop being gay. As a gay man, it only makes sense for me to be in a gay relationship. When you cast a shadow of shame over my relationship, I will once again feel shame and a sense of rejection.

The LGBT community is the only minority group to experience the pain of rejection by family for being who they are. It is a basic human need to feel accepted by family. I know my brother loves me. He may even say that he accepts me. By not accepting my relationship, he is still making me feel like I am "OTHER". Like I am deeply flawed and living a life of perversion. It's a continuation of the thread of shame that has run through my life, leaving me damaged.

Like all LGBT people, I must make my way through all of the stages of shame in life. The stages of shame are denial, acceptance and authenticity. I will continue to fight the toxic, bigoted ideologies that have held my community down. It is my hope that one day gay children can grow up free from the pain of shame and rejection. May they grow up with a sense of peace and authenticity that has eluded many generations before them. When someone asks "Are you gay", may there not be 25 years before finally answering "Yes I am!" Better yet... may the question not be asked because it's okay to be gay.

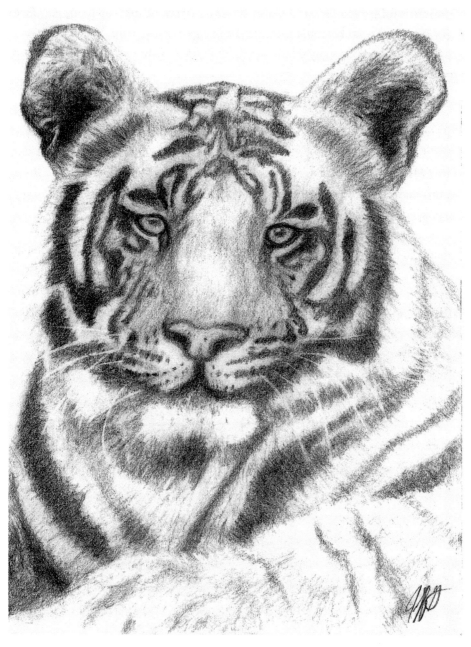

TIGER
Jeff Gysbers

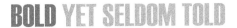

My Story

By Robert Siltman

Hello. My name is Robert Siltman, and these are some of my truths. I don't like to use the word "story" because that sounds fictional, and these are things you cannot make up. So, welcome to the mess that is my life. Where does one even begin to reflect on a lifetime of mental health issues, traumas, and addictions. To choose only a few brief months of time is like choosing grains of sand off the beach. This is my life and more washes up each day.

I am the oldest of three children. We grew up with very little money. My folks were always gone working or at the bar. We were left home, unsupervised. However, there was always food on the table and we had clothes on our backs. The old man drove truck, so we rarely saw him except when he returned and whooped my ass for everything that was done while he was away. Because I was the oldest, I was responsible. Thus a vicious cycle began of being thrown through walls and beaten up with anything that could be picked up, so as to "make me tough." Looking back, I realize this is probably why I started using drugs at such a young age. It was my attempt to escape the reality that was my life. I started with whatever was at hand, tobacco, booze and marijuana. Around the time I was seven, I was into cocaine and anything I could do to escape. I ran away with a carnival when I was 15, and my drug use escalated using meth, LSD and crack cocaine. It was then I saw my first shooting—a drive-by right in front of me. I will never forget the sound of gunshots ringing out or seeing the people fall down. I was walking to the store in Memphis, Tennessee. Three people were gunned down and all I could do was run.

About a month later I was sitting in Coffee County Jail in Douglas, Georgia. I was busted in a hotel raid and charged with possession of crack cocaine. Georgia is nothing like Minnesota. They still had chain gangs and guards didn't come on the jail block. Me, being a Yankee and a white boy made for a truly rough stay, and that's an understatement. I sat there for almost 14 months before I broke down and called home for bail money. I returned to Minnesota and moved in with a friend and his girl. It was a hostile environment. One night while drunk, of course, we went for a drive. We ended up rolling the car, end over end and side to side. My friend was ejected. After crawling out of the car and finding him with his head split open, I held his head together while someone stopped and called 911. He lived, but suffered brain trauma. A few months later I was still living with them. We didn't slow anything down and they got into a nasty fight. I left and passed out in the car. My friend came, took off in the car, and hit a telephone pole at 90 mph. I was thrown through the windshield, peeling my face up and causing a traumatic brain injury. I only remember bits and pieces of the incident.

After healing from the accident, I met Miss Molly, fell in love and moved to St. Cloud. Everything was going great. She got pregnant and we were ecstatic. Sadly, this was not meant to be as our son was born prematurely. Initially he was doing well, but he became sick before we could bring him home. We were told if he did pull through, he would be severely disabled, leaving us with a choice no parent should have to make. I held our son in my arms as he died.

I then returned to drugs–hard. I wasn't able to forget or forgive myself, and I still haven't. We had another child, a daughter, who was healthy and beautiful. I was too far gone in drugs and self-pity to realize what a miracle she was. I spiraled even further down, wanting only oblivion. I threw away everything good in my life, including Molly and my daughter. I was back in the jail system, homeless and living in a tent. A friend found me and offered me a job with the railroad making good money. I felt on top of the world and so fed my habit, using meth all day and drinking all night. On one of my days off, a girl I was seeing and I decided to go to a bar at Piney Ridge Resort. This ended badly with my first stint in prison. I was assaulted by the police, tazed multiple times and then got "the boots" after being handcuffed. I reported it, but there was no squad video. I was bruised and could hardly move for weeks. Even though this was my first felony, the judge sent me straight to prison for 33 months. After being released, I remember how hard it was to return to "normal" life. There was no help, no programs, nothing, just "Here's your little $100 gate feel and see ya!" Having nothing and nowhere to go made it easy to return to the drug life and night lights.

Two years later I was back in trouble. I caught a pedifile with two underage girls, ages 9 and 14. I did what I believed was right and stopped him from damaging those girls further. Turns out the law saw it differently and I was given an 81 month sentence for burglary and 1st degree assault. The judge took pity on me because of the circumstances and gave me probation. I tried really hard to do good. I met my angel, Stacy, and she brought me back from the brink of destruction. She was my high school sweetheart and it was definitely like a fairytale. She sobered me up, helped me to heal and become a happy family man. I stayed clean and sober for a few years, but this was also not meant to be my happily ever after. One evening I was working on a roof when we talked for the last time. Man, I wish I knew then that it was the last time. I have so many unfinished things I would say. I finished work and went to where we were supposed to meet and she wasn't there. I tried calling–nothing. As I was waiting I got a call that there had been a terrible plane crash and I just knew. I ran the couple miles to town, but it was too late. She was already gone. The only way to identify her was by her tattoos.

For months I tried to hold it together for the kids, but after the funeral I just wasn't strong enough. Booze and drugs took over my life. The more I hated myself, the more I used. Back in and out of the system over the next couple years, I met my now ex-wife, whom I loved. But, it was a using relationship. We had kids but lost them because of our drug use, yet used more because we lost them. Our relationship was strained because I couldn't get over my past and grieve or heal. I know this was unfair to my wife. I ended up executing my sentence, not for new crimes, but because I couldn't stay sober.

This time I did my time right. I was the perfect inmate, got let out on early work release and got a great job. I completed a year of work release with no issues. I had high hopes, but without any kind of treatment, I just couldn't stay sober after I was released, which leads me to where I am now. I have been sitting close to a year in jail, trying to get the help I desperately need. I am on medication, am working on and off with mental health professions, and hopefully will get the treatment I need. But, there are so many roadblocks when you are incarcerated. Most people cannot get the proper help they need and deserve while they are here. I have seen many improvements during my life of incarceration. Jail staff, medical staff and mental health has definitely advanced by leaps and bounds. However, the courts and probation have deteriorated to a slow, sluggish entity dragging thousands of souls chained to them in their wake. I write my story to let it be seen and to help break those chains that bind us to the past's archaic ways so people like me can get the help they need and deserve. No one should be left behind, lost and forgotten because of their addictions.

This is my story and there are many like it. I hope with all my heart that it becomes a success story so I can help others like me who struggle with addiction to just know they are not alone.

To be continued . . .

Victim No More

By Waasumockwe

Aaniin/Boozhoo:
Niigaaniiwaasumookwe Nindizhnikaans, Michele Berger Indigoo, Makwa Dodem, Chiminising Nindoonjibaa.

I said Hello/Greetings:

My name is "She comes with the Lightning." I am also called Michele Berger. I am a member of the Bear Clan and my hometown is Isle, MN. I gave a traditional Mille Lacs Anishinaabe greeting, as I do verbally when I greet an audience when I speak on panels, or as an invited speaker.

As I said, I grew up and went to school in Isle, Mn where I lived with my family two miles from town. We were known as some of the "poor Indians" who were even less than any of our Native American relatives because the "ones with money" were also sober, working class, and church going, and the children were athletic. That gave them an edge of popularity and acceptance.

I had to work hard in my classes and was on the honor roll all through my high school years and even lettered in Volleyball, Softball and Basketball. But because I was one of the "out group," my academic and athletic performances were overlooked. No matter how hard I tried, how pleasant I was to others, I could not shake the label that hung over my head like a dark cloud. That level of oppression did something to me that I still have trouble acknowledging. Instead of internalizing and falling into a depressive state, I grew angry and began using alcohol and drugs and was extremely antagonistic in my reverse racism. I stole from, threatened and fought people to get what I wanted, and I justified my actions by remembering the treatment I received when I was in grade school. Having been labeled as dirty, stupid, poor, ugly, and lower class made me want to prove people wrong. I excelled in most areas, but that did nothing in the town to improve their view of me. Knowing my children would also endure this, I decided to move out of the area.

I moved my children to Brainerd and we began receiving the same treatment here! My kids were singled out in school when it came to discipline, there was a lack of exposure to their own culture, and staff played favorites with other students in sports and games. I tried to overlook that and encouraged my kids to hang with "our own kind." I also applied for a job and house, as we were staying with family members. We did not qualify for certain housing programs. Others saw my "public assistance" income or my tribal per capita payment, and I could see the dismissal coming.

I believe we were and still are followed around local stores, being watched for theft and suspicious activity. While I did such things in the past, I have since seen the error of my ways and will go without before I would steal again. Our landlord tried many times to legally remove us from his property, as we only became eligible due to some extreme family crisis. (The father of my children was declared officially missing for 3 months and then found deceased, so our family was moved to the top of the program waiting list). The landlord later declined our request for help and to move from our unit after a flood destroyed our personal belongings. He installed an air conditioner in the apartment and made me get an account at his electric company (with no previous notice but a demand/ultimatum that if I did not comply we would have to leave). We had another flood (due to faulty heat registers) and he only replaced the carpet. So we put up with some substandard housing for five years before I was eligible to purchase a home. Even some of the property management and realty companies would refuse to work with me and my family.

I began going to school at Central Lakes College and working for my tribe, learning different ways to be healthy and happy. I am also in therapy to address my anger issues, to learn coping skills and deal with childhood trauma. With all the exposure to equity and inclusion in various local committees and boards, I took it on myself to work with allies and advocates in the area. I am also taking courses on race, ethnicity and oppression, intercultural communication and many other similar classes in the Human Services Program. This has given me tools to look at my own racial identity, challenge my biases and see where I can also improve my cultural competence.

I am now an advocate for my People, my family, my neighbors and any other group of people who need assistance finding their voice. I have found a wonderful group of people who share this view and are action-oriented, not just willing to talk about it. From the 100 conversations, to various meetings, conferences, panels and discussions, local pow-wow and cultural events, I feel I have a strong place in my community and want my children to see that change is possible. We just have to find the right people with the motivation and desire to change and work with them.

Miigwech bizindaan. (Thank you for listening/reading).

Meth

By Devon Jotham
AKA Kirk Nelson

Meth, you are stupid.
You're a life-killing fool.
Why did you take me to hell where you come
from?
Why did you take my family, friends, and
loved ones?

You've made me turn my back on everything
that means anything to me.
You've made me feel like death.

Meth, from this day forward, you have no
hold on me.
I rebuke you.
My God has died so that you will be
removed from me.
My God will destroy you.
You have no more hold on my life.

There's nothing good that you have ever
done.
I pray that you will die to every one.
You're nothing to me.
Die. Die. Die.
Die, because I love my family.
They're worth more than you!

Jesse's Story

By Jesse Bell

Growing up on a 100 acre farm in eastern Oregon, I knew what hard work was at an early age. Like most farm kids there were chores before and after school and weekends. My mom and dad were alcoholic addicts. My real dad, who left when I was three, was a coke dealer. My parents would drink in front of me but usually tried to hide the pot, coke and crank. As I got older, about 7 or 8, I knew. My stepdad drilled it into me that what happens at home stays at home. He was an abusive drunk verbally and physically to my mom and often verbally abusive to me.

The summer before my freshman year my mom finally had enough and we moved to a nearby town with her new boyfriend. I don't think he used drugs but was a drinker. He and my mom were always at the bars.

I was very shy and had low self esteem so making new friends was very hard. Luckily the neighbor kid was my age and he made sure I didn't get in with the wrong crowd—the "good" kids. Needless to say I was going to parties, drinking and smoking weed.

By the time I graduated we moved three times. Three new boyfriends, three new towns and three new schools. I was always getting in with the wrong crowd but made a lot of friends. When I was 19 I moved back to my home town, got a full time job and an apartment. Still drinking and smoking weed. By the time I was 21 I was married, had a daughter and divorced. Later I signed my parental rights over to my ex.

One night I was having a party and a buddy asked me if I wanted to do a line. I thought it was coke so I snorted a line. WOW! It wasn't coke, it was crank. A couple hours later I smoked some off a foil. It felt amazing. A couple hours after that I shot up for the first time and was hooked.

The next three years was one big party. When I was 25 I met my second wife. She was going to college to be an RN. She drank and that was it. She was not cool with me doing drugs at all. The more we were together the less crank and weed I used. After a couple of months all I did was drink—a lot. Within a year we were married and soon after that she was pregnant with our daughter. At this point I was smoking weed behind her back. By the time our daughter was four I was back to using crank. My wife, six months pregnant, moved to Brainerd MN where she is from and filed for divorce.

The next two years I fell hard. My mom died of alcoholism and I was too high to go to the funeral. I caught a third degree assault and misdemeanor drug possession charge and ended up in treatment. My ex contacted me. We start talking daily and decided after treatment that I should move to Brainerd.

In 2000 I moved and within six months I was smoking weed again. Shortly after that I tried crystal meth for the first time. It was a more intense high than crank and lasted longer. I started doing lines every day. I would limit myself and not use after three PM so I could eat a big dinner and get a decent night's sleep. I had a fulltime job, a house, and newer vehicles. I was a functional addict and my wife didn't know.

In 2004 our second son, third child, was born. Around mid-year 2006, my wife started going out to bars after work at 11 PM. By 2007 she found a new man and we split up for good. Now I couldn't afford my meth habit so I started selling to few friends to pay for my personal use. I still had my job and saw my kids on a regular basis. Within a year she lost her job due to drinking and moved to Apple Valley with our kids. Needless to say, I didn't get to see my kids that much. I started using more and running around at night getting very little sleep. I started shooting up again. A few months of this and I got fired for being late and sometimes not showing up for work at all. My work offered to pay for treatment and I refused. What a dumb ass I was. It was the best job I ever had.

The next five years I was a fulltime drug dealer. I sold mostly meth but also weed and pills. I paid my bills, had a place to stay, and saw my kids once every couple of months. I wasn't only addicted to meth but to the money too. I liked the attention, everybody wanted me and if they had money or something to trade, I was there. Driving around every day slinging meth.

In 2014 I get busted. Second degree sale and third degree possession. I went to jail and my house gets raided. What the cops didn't find my "friends" took. Luckily nobody found my money stash buried in the back yard so I was able to hire an attorney, and charges were reduced to third degree sale and fourth degree possession. I had 20 years probation and 42 months prison time hanging over my head. Six months later I had two urine analyses that were dirty which led to outpatient treatment. I was kicked out for using and that led to 30 days of inpatient treatment. I lasted four days and then got high.

I was with my third wife now for a few months but not married yet. In early 2015 I started going to Crystal Meth Anonymous (CMA) groups. I could make it a week, sometimes two, but would then relapse. I was always welcomed back to CMA with open arms. No judging, no dirty looks, just a lot of hugs and friendly faces.

June 25, 2016, was my last relapse. I was home and locked in my bathroom, tired of being sick and tired, the lies and deception, I slammed about a gram and a half. What happened next I can't explain. The next thing I know I'm flushing the rest of my dope down the toilet. I wasn't even high, just really confused. What just happened?

I honestly believe that God had a different plan for me. I just celebrated seven years free from meth and 10 years from alcohol.

I've been chairing the CMA meeting at the Up Front Alano Club in Brainerd for six years now. I am a sponsor and mentor. I carry the CMA message whenever I can. We are even going to be in an upcoming parade.

I have an amazing wife who hasn't left my side through the lies and relapses. We have a nice house on 10 acres and nice things and cars. I've rebuilt the relationship with my three kids and have two grandsons and a great job. I can look in the mirror and smile back at myself.

I owe it all to God and my CMA family.

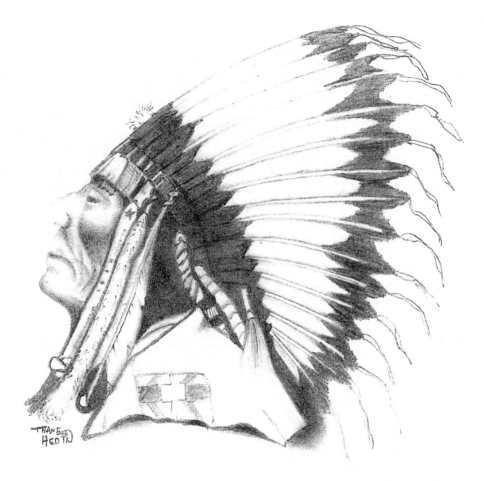

INDIAN CHIEF
Thane Hedin

Shane Holmin

By Shane Holmin

I wanted to start of by thanking you for the opportunity to share my story. I often say my life is an open book and in sharing my story it may help someone in some way who may possibly be going through the same thing. I knew I was gay from a very young age and was always too afraid to admit who I was due to how society and my religion portrayed homosexuals. As an adolescent I tried my hardest to hide the real me deep inside and tried to conform and fit into what society's standards labeled as a real man. Years went by and the bullying got worse. I tried not to let it affect me since to the bullies it was just their assumptions of me. I kept my head up and just kept moving forward.

My story begins with my move to rural Minnesota and still being in the closet. I met someone and that someone happened to be a woman. We just clicked, and although knowing I was gay, I thought maybe it would pass because the connection we had and love we shared was so strong. I ended up making that woman my wife and we started a family and had 2 beautiful children. We had an amazing relationship and felt that nothing could break us.

At age 23 is where my struggles began. I had a male friend and tried to fit into being heteronormative. We would go fishing, hunting and talk about cars. He was my best friend. We had gone to a concert and he dropped me off at my car. As I was getting out he said, "What, don't I get a kiss?" I laughed and called him crazy, and we went our own ways. On my drive home my mind started racing and all these feelings I had pushed away resurfaced.

I needed to be honest with myself and with my wife. I walked into the house and told my wife we needed to talk. She looked at me and said, "You're gay." I was shocked and taken back but mustered up the courage to answer honestly and I replied "Yes." We had a long talk. My wife stated she had thought about my gayness, but figured because of our bond and love we could work through this because people work through a lot harder things in life. She told me she was sorry I couldn't be my true self for all these years. We remain to this day best friends and still celebrate all the holidays as a family.

Now at 23 I'm an openly gay man with 2 children. Living in this small town becomes hard and the bullying got worse not only for myself but for my kids as well. So I made the decision to move to Minneapolis. It was a dark time for me, and I tried to take my own life.

Then at 25 I needed/wanted to be closer to my kids and made the move back to northern Minnesota where I started a 4-H group and became a Boy Scout leader and got involved with a lot of school events. I felt the locals of this area were not welcoming, and I feel would go out of their way to make sure I knew "My Kind" was not accepted here. I had signs put in my yard on multiple occasions that had the words faggot and queer on them. Men and women in passing while at the grocery store would make derogatory comments, but I just tried to keep my head high and ignore the ignorance.

Co-workers went as far as to spread rumors that I was operating a gay sex farm and it's the only reason why I was involved in Boy Scouts and 4-H was to be around young boys. One co-worker also happened to be a mother of one of my Boy Scouts. She had been in my home multiple times and I thought she was a friend. When the authorities got involved, she tried to deny she knew me. At that time, I and another gay Scout leader (female) were asked to step down from our positions.

I have been physically attacked and had derogatory slurs yelled at me when visiting downtown in an adjacent city for being openly gay. My kids were bullied, and their classmates would say things about them having a faggot for a dad and other ignorant things. It got hard for them. My daughter hit a dark spot in her life to the point she became a cutter and wanted to end her life.

My kids went to a rural school and they promote a Zero Tolerance on bullying but as a parent I found that not to be true. We were called to the high school because of a bullying incident between my daughter and another student. At this meeting my daughter stated her side and that this kid would not lay off her and would say and write things to her about her gay dad. The teacher admitted to knowing this had been going on for a while but didn't do anything about it until my daughter had reach her breaking point.

Now I am in the part of my life that I have decided to become active, and not let people silence me. I found a local nonprofit called Project Rainbow and became a board member. This group truly saved my life and gave me a positive outlet as a gay man. Other opportunities started presenting themselves. I was asked by the high school and the college to discussing my story and LGBTQ+

issues with the classrooms. That then turned into a mentoring opportunity at The Shop for the LGBQ+ youth for Rainbow Road. It became my passion, and I also became a Kinship Partner. If my story could be heard and change the life of even one LGBTQ+ community member, that's a success to me.

Current day I remain active in all these things mentioned above and am always open to or seeking new opportunities to continue to spread awareness for the LGBQ+ community. I often get asked how I continue to live in the area and my response is "I've had to fight way too hard to become comfortable in my own skin and to make a name for myself and ill be dammed if I'm going to let ignorance drive me away." That and finding the people who see and support me for me.

My story is much longer with way more details but so this didn't become a novel I tried my best to shorten it. I thank you again for this opportunity to share my story and am always open to further conversation.

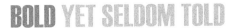

Why?

By Alvin

Alvin grew up on a farm where life was all church, work, and school and his father was quite harsh. Being a workaholic was the expectation, and criticism was the norm.

In grade school, because of poor handwriting due to shaky hands, his 2nd grade teacher made him wear a wire brace. That was his first experience of feeling different from others. Much later in life Alvin found out that his teacher had also suggested counseling for anxiety. No one ever talked about that.

Then in 5th grade Alvin scored in the 95th percentile in the Iowa Basic Skills testing, 98th percentile in Science and 97th in Math. A lot of expectations were placed on him because of the high scores. Everyone talked about that.

Marijuana became a welcome friend at age 15; it did something really good for him. Using pot several times a day throughout high school became the norm. In spite of this, or perhaps because of this, high school came easy for him. He got good grades, without ever taking a book home, he was President of the Northern Division of the Minnesota Association of Student Councils his Junior Year, ran the District Convention, and took part in three State conventions and two National conventions. He also participated in Speech, Band, Drama and Cross Country.

A life dream was to spend 20 years in the Army so he joined right after high school. That did not work out; neither did several jobs and marriage. He didn't understand why.

Despite alcohol always making him sick, he decided he needed to learn to drink because he was going into the Army. Alcohol would become the only drug that caused problems in his life, and it caused a lot. Going through Drug and Alcohol treatment at age 20 helped with sobriety for about 7 months. The next 14-15 years he was in and out of 12-Step meetings like Alcoholics Anonymous and was never able to achieve 7 months again until the age of 35 when he had an adjustment of his attitude about God. Twelve Step groups gave him permission to seek his own understanding of God. He currently has 28 years of sobriety.

He decided to return to college in his late 30's, thinking lack of education was why he hadn't been successful. In spite of having excellent grades, he had difficulty getting much done, had dizziness and fatigue, and, again, didn't know why.

Medical professionals were the next step. Several physical tests were completed and all came back negative. Finally someone suggested taking the MMPI, which he told them would be a waste of time. The one thing he knew wasn't wrong with him was his psychological state. Then the diagnosis came back —Panic Disorder with Depression and Agoraphobia. This was the first step in learning the "Why."

Seeing a psychiatrist for a year and doing many drug trials did not work out well. He switched to a psychologist for a year. He saw both for the next four years, and the correct anti-depressant was finally discovered, which he continues to take today.

Within a few credits of obtaining a degree in Organizational Management and Communication, he just couldn't finish. He applied for Social Security Disability and was approved on the third try. When the Judge declared him 100% disabled at the hearing, it was exactly what he wanted to hear but possibly the most difficult thing he ever had to hear.

Being married and divorced three times in early adulthood was discouraging; however, he did marry again. He was feeling somewhat better and had found a community in church.

His health worsened. He didn't leave home for several years except for doctor's visits and brief shopping trips. His weight climbed to 250 pounds, and he had headaches that lasted 24 hours with pain so severe it caused vomiting. Intestinal cramping plagued him at night for several years. The VA put him on a high dose of Clonazepam (a Benzodiazepine) 3 times a day for 2.5 years. He would come to find out it was the most physically addictive drug he had ever been involved with.

Then his "Shawshank Redemption" moment came, "You need to get busy living or get busy dying." He chose living and decided to make three changes:

1)   Medicine – He discontinued the Clonazepam and after a full 20 years of abstinence from Cannabis, he started using it as a medicine which he would come to believe saved his life.

2) Diet – Working on an Elimination Diet helped him figure out what was making him sick. He found that fiber and less-processed foods were good for him and ultra-processed foods were not. He stopped drinking calories with the exception of milk. Salty and sugary snacks were replaced with fruit, berries and nuts. The goal was not to lose weight, just to feel better. Ultimately 100 pounds came off and stayed off.

3) People he hung around with. – After the first two changes made such a difference, he knew he needed community, to be around people. Church had left him feeling judged. In frustration over who the Fundamentalist Christians thought was "Their Guy," he typed, "Jesus is a Liberal" into the Search Bar of his phone and ended up at the United Church of Christ website which led to the First Congregational United Church of Christ in Brainerd. He went the next Sunday and had a hard time getting out of his vehicle because it seemed as if the door handle was too heavy. After several minutes he was able to get it open and go in. Since then he tells people that they've made his door handle lighter.

An unfortunate outcome of changing people he hung around with was another divorce.

For years the tape that played over and over in his head was "I don't feel good." Then one day on his way home from church he noticed it was "I feel good!" Between church and 12-step groups such as Alcoholics Anonymous, the importance of community became very real.

Working with other organizations has been so beneficial. In the back yard of the Up Front Alano Club, a Recovery Garden was started in cooperation with the United Church of Christ, The Up Front Alano Club and Crow Wing Energized. He is proud and grateful to be a part of that.

As Alvin says, "When I pray about my struggles, God distracts me by presenting me with opportunities to help others. That has made such a positive difference. My most common prayer is that I may be of use to my God and my fellows." He also says, "The miracle isn't that God is going to 'fix me.' The miracle is that God is going to make use of me to help others in spite of my disabilities."

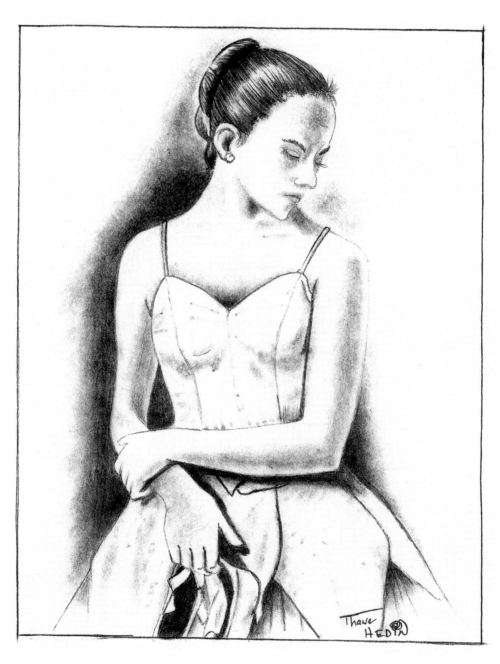

WEDDING GIRL
Thane Hedin

A Poem for Sid

By Sid Salem

There's someone I would love to see
But I know she'd first want me
    to work on me
For the first time in my life
I'm glad I'm not on dope
For the first time in my life
I've got a glimpse of hope

So many times I've done myself
    tremendous harm
From smoking or snorting or
    sticking a needle in my arm
I'm learning to make up for the mistakes
    I've made in the past
I'm learning a new way to live
    with pain that won't last
Every night though,
    I think of her in my head
And I think of every word that she has said

I know I'll be locked up for
    an indefinite while
But I know when I get out
    I'll see her smile
I know I'm making progress
    to a better life
And I see how much happier
    I am becoming in every strife
This new life I want to live
    I want to live
    I'll definitely see this through
But for now, I bid thee farewell
    And adieu

A Mother's Journey

By Barbara Flynn McColgan

We all have times in our lives when we must do something that we find difficult, that we'd rather avoid. That was the case in the summer of 2012 when an attempt by some to amend the Minnesota constitution to define marriage as only being between one man and one woman resulted in this measure being put on the ballot for the people to vote on in November. I knew I would Vote NO, but as the mother of a gay son, I also knew it was critical that a majority of my family, friends, and neighbors voted NO as well. So, I participated in a training with Outfront Minnesota, a group that works for LGBTQIA+ equality, and officially became part of the VOTE NO Campaign. That meant talking to people, lots and lots of people, and not just "easy to talk to" people. The local United Congregational Church allowed us to use a meeting room in their building as a base for our phone calling. We began calling people on the voter lists they gave us, total strangers, strangers with all sorts of different attitudes and beliefs on the subject. We had a script we followed that didn't talk about civil rights and equality, but rather required us to share our personal experiences and asked voters about their experiences with LGBTQIA+ folks as well.

Up until that point in my almost 60 years of life I had not been politically active. I'd never helped with campaigning or done calling, and I found it frightening. I had to talk with a lot of different people as part of my job, but this was totally different. This was EXTREMELY IMPORTANT!! It was for my son!! I found a quote from Eleanor Roosevelt that became my mantra. "Do one thing every day that scares you!" Little did I know when I started out that just a month before election day, due to her health concerns, I would have to step in and take over for the local coordinator to keep our efforts going right up until election day. Now that REALLY scared me, but it had to be done.

I had lived in Brainerd for 37 years at that point and I knew a lot of people but talking to folks about something so "controversial" was a new experience.

Before each call I would take a deep breath, tell myself "You can do this," and dial. The types of responses I got were as varied as the crowds at the Crow Wing County Fair. Some listened with interest and wanted to discuss the proposed amendment, while others said rude, cruel, or unkind things and quickly hung up. Some responses surprised me, in both positive and negative ways. There was the woman in her 90s who asked, "Why can't we just let people live their lives in whatever way makes them happy?" or the people who seemed to grow and change their opinion as you were talking to them. The hardest conversations for me were those with friends or people I knew well, when I wrongly assumed they would agree that this amendment would be bad for Minnesotans and should not pass, only to find out that they supported the proposed amendment. I think I "put on my armor" when calling strangers but let my guard down when talking to friends. The negative responses and lack of understanding really hurt, especially when we were specifically talking about MY SON who they knew well!! After stating how personal and important this was to my son and my family, I was absolutely confounded by the reply, "Well, if it passes this will hurt people who don't support gay marriage too!!" Now, ten years after same sex marriage became legal, I would really like to go back and ask them how they have been hurt, or how their lives have been changed. I couldn't help but wonder if their opinions would change if or when they might learn that they had a gay relative or even a gay grandchild in their family.

Minnesota became the only state to defeat an anti-same sex marriage amendment by popular vote and went on in the spring of 2013 to pass legislation making same sex marriage legal in our state. We were all overjoyed!!

This campaign was implemented at a very grassroots level. It showed me that every individual CAN make a difference, and it is important for us to all do our part. This experience showed me that I can do things that scare me, and I can do important things. It made me proud to be a Minnesotan. Sadly, it also showed me that there are still too many people out there who lack empathy and kindness. Most importantly, it gave me the chance to make many new friends, and to watch them experience, some for the first time, unconditional acceptance. I knew it was a journey worth traveling. We had done the right thing.

Tony's Story

By Jim Newgord

In the early seventy's my wife Elizabeth (Itty) and I had just started our married lives together. We lived in Sauk Rapids, Minnesota where Itty was a special education teacher dealing with the early education of young handicapped children. That was where we first came in contact with Tony, who would become our adopted son.

Through Itty's work we would host Tony at our house periodically. He was two years old and would stay with us for up to several days. Tony was a sweet boy who we took an instant liking to. He was always there to help. I was called upon to play Santa Claus for the center's Christmas party. When it came time to pass out presents to the children Tony was right there to hand me presents and then deliver them to the other kids.

He took some effort in the care area, due to an injury he experienced at the hands of his father, he had a trac, (a hole in his throat that enabled to breath.) The trac had be cleaned out several times a day so he could breathe normally. He also had not been potty trained at this time.

At this time we had purchased a small farm south of Brainerd. We moved and just about the time we got relocated Tony's social worker called. He asked us if we would be interested in taking Tony as a foster child with the hopes that we would adopt him.

We agreed and two weeks later we were parents. The challenges began shortly. The school district informed us that there was no early childhood education program available. Itty did her research and not only got all the information that she wanted, but also secured a spot on the Region 5 Board to initiate a program to address the needs of zero- to five-year-old children. But when we called to register Tony, we were informed that the class was full. I was on the phone with one of the program teachers and I told her that Tony had an IEP (individual education plan,) and that the school system was compelled to offer services. There was dead silence on the phone for a short period and we were given a time and place to start in the "prep program."

During Tony's younger years in school we ran into things that most parents never have to experience. There were many times that Tony would get home from school and spend the evening sulking or crying because of the way other kids were treating him. He was constantly the target of name calling. He had more than once during those years told us that he was going out on stage in front of the whole school and stab himself that would make the other kids sorry they treated him that way.

Another thing that happened during school was the definition for kids with special needs was changed and he was mainstreamed. This presented a problem because of his difficulties in math and history. We spent hours with him working on his studies and trying to get him ready for tests. After a couple of years the definition changed back and he was once again placed on special needs status. Despite all the adversity we experienced, Tony graduated from high school.

Challenges in school were just part of our story; another was medical expenses. One of the reoccurring problems Tony experienced was an infected shunt—a tube that ran from his head to his stomach to drain off excess spinal fluid. During his growth the tube would become too short and as a result the tube would get infected. With all of his health concerns we couldn't afford health insurance, so the state continued taking care of his insurance.

Raising an adopted child with special needs can have other unexpected twists and turns. We got to the point of finalizing the adoption when Tony was six. During the time Tony was growing and we set boundaries and rules for him like keep your room picked up and take out the garbage etc. If he didn't want to do something he would tell us we were not his real parents and he didn't have to listen to us. After all, his real parents wouldn't treat him this way.

We were told at one of the adoptive parents' workshops that this was a common ploy of adoptive children. We called his social worker and asked her what we could do. Part of the adoption was that we were not, under any circumstances, to tell Tony about his biological parents and the reasons that he was up for adoption. The social worker set up an appointment to visit with Tony without us present. After the meeting the social worker said she found it necessary to tell him the circumstances of his adoption. She let him know that his father was in prison and his mother was a problem drinker and he was so fortunate to have us as his adoptive parents. After that we never heard him complain again.

And the adventure continues...

Tracy's Story

By Tracy Lamb

I have traveled a long and challenging road my whole life. My parents, once married, were divorced when I was born. Shortly after my birth, I became deathly ill and, thank God, ended up at the University of Minnesota Hospital. I had lost my digestive fluids which meant I had been getting poisoned from the inside out. I later came to believe that my biological mother had been feeding me spoiled milk intending to harm me.

A few months later, my biological mother left me at the babysitter's house to go on a date and she never came back. My biological mother didn't want me. My Uncle Harry, himself having gone through abandonment as a child, wanted to take me in. But Social Services placed me in foster care.

My foster care parents, Dorothy and Alfred DeCent, were great people who embraced and cared for me with unconditional love. I learned to return that same kind of love to them. Eventually, my father was granted full custody of me. I remember it like it was yesterday. When Social Services came to take me away, I looked up at Dorothy and Alfred and pleaded, "I will be a good girl. Don't let them take me away!" I'm sure it broke their hearts and, somehow, they maintained partial custody of me until I was ten. At that point, my dad was legally able to stop them from having any contact and that left me a broken-hearted little girl.

From age four until about eleven, I lived with my father but was frequently removed and placed in protective care. When my dad gained custody of me, his wife and her daughter moved out. I think he blamed me for his wife leaving him. When I was ten years old, my biological mother told me that a Native American man may have been my real biological father. She wasn't sure. Even as a child, that possibility made sense to me as it could explain why my siblings were all blonde-haired, light complected, and had hazel eyes. I, on the other hand, was dark complected, had medium dark hair and brown eyes. That could explain, also, why the man who was raising me seemed so angry and punishing toward me. He may have suspected that he wasn't really my dad. From that time on, I began to study the culture of Indigenous people. I liked what I learned and in my own simple way began to mold my thoughts and actions as an Indigenous person might.

During my pre-teen years, at one point, my dad had to spend six-nine months in jail. Going to live with my Uncle Harry in another city, forced me to leave the friends and place I had come to love. Prior to this relocation, I had been a straight "A" student, never missed a day of school, attending even if I was sick. Teachers had to make me go home. I loved school. Starting sixth grade in the new town, just having been torn from the only parent I had, I was devastated. My reaction was to slowly start rebelling against everyone, even my Uncle Harry, whom I adored. My grades fell to even less than a "C" average. I started to hang out with the wrong crowd. The only good thing about the move was that I learned my foster mom, Dorothy DeCent, was living in a nearby nursing home. Nobody was going to stop me from visiting her, so every day after school, I detoured through her room.

After six months in jail, my dad was released and I was returned to his care. That's when the little rebel in me went full force. I ran the streets at night, my grades fell to complete "D" and "F" level. I continued to visit my foster mom as often as I could. I got into alcohol and drugs. I just didn't care. I was sexually assaulted when I was twelve and had a still-born child. That didn't help my lost little world. At age thirteen, I was diagnosed with manic depression.

By the time I was fourteen, I was totally out of anyone's control. Things got worse when my foster mom died and my dad wouldn't let me go to the funeral. He said, "They are NOT your family!" But they were the only real "family" I had ever known. In two years' time, I lost my foster mom, then foster dad and finally my biological grandpa. But, unknown to me, the tables were starting to turn. On the night before my grandpa died, I promised him that if I was still doing any drugs, I would quit by my eighteenth birthday. At the time of his death, I already expected to be dead before my eighteenth birthday. I had literally been doing all the alcohol and drugs with the hope of leaving this world. I wanted to die. The only three people in my life who loved me unconditionally were now all gone. I didn't die. On my eighteenth birthday, I quit doing drugs.

I was sent to Port Group Home for Girls. It was there I met a cook that we all called "Grandma Cindy." She sat me down and asked about my life. She hugged me and said, "Only you can change the outcome in your life." Another

Port worker told me that if I could progress through the trust levels there, they would find me a job. I worked hard at keeping the rules, and soon was employed as a janitor at Harrison School. Next, I went to work at Goodwill where I met Kathy, my supervisor - a great boss and a great person. At Port, I worked up to Level 2, with a couple of hiccups, but stayed there. I was looking forward to Level 3. I got to go on a weekend visit with my dad. I told him I had a job and had a lot of money saved. Two weeks before Level 3 graduation, my dad pulled me out of Port. Maybe it was to gain access to my money. Who knows? When I got back home, I went back to my old ways, not drinking, but now smoking pot for the next two years. I was so crushed that I had not made it to Level 3. It felt like my hard work had just been ripped from me. By eighteen, I was working and on my own. I kept the promise I made to my grandfather about quitting drug use, but was drinking again and going to parties.

My life changed dramatically when I hit twenty. I became pregnant with my daughter. Her father was a Native American. Having grown up the way I did, I wanted things to be better for my child. So, no more alcohol. After her birth, I got pregnant again but miscarried. A sad day. Then I got pregnant with my son. I did my best as a young mom. I worked hard to support them while suffering in an abusive relationship with their father. The last straw came when my children were age three, and, one-and-a-half. My partner nearly killed me. "Why," you might ask, "did you stay with him for three years?" I so desperately wanted my children, unlike my own experience, to have two parents in their home. Having been abused as a child, my partner's abuse of me almost seemed normal. God helped me that day as my little ones miraculously enabled my escape. By this time, having been exposed to Mormon, Salvation Army, Baptist, and Native American spirituality, I believe in the Christian God and in the Indigenous people's Gitchi Manitou, Creator. Maybe the same.

After escaping my partner's wrath, I raised my children on my own. Having missed graduation because of my daughter's birth, I went back to high school and graduated two years late, 1997. I attended Central Lakes College, Brainerd, and earned a degree in photography. For the past seven years, I have been employed at Central Lakes Drug Testing and love my work. I aspire to someday owning the company. Today, I am grandma to three beautiful girls.

Here's what I'd like to say to whomever reads my story. I had a few inspirational people in my life. They helped me get through some very rough times. I was truly a lost soul. Why didn't God take care of me as an infant? Why did I go through so much hurt in life? What was my purpose here? I found my purpose through my current job. My purpose is to help others. Many people helped me and now I can help others. With love and support from strangers, good friends and family members, your story, like mine, can move in a positive and enduring direction.

There is one person, now deceased, to whom I owe my newfound confidence. This counselor pushed me from hiding in my house, alone and dejected, into seeing new possibilities, and doing the work necessary to grow into them. Sometimes all we need to do is talk to someone. To my friend, therapist J.P. Whalen, I say, "Thank you for the five years you invested in helping me to heal, hope, grow, and find joy." He would have said, "No, you did it on your own." Thanks also to all the other guardian angels mentioned in my story, and to community members who shared food with us when we were children, teachers and professors who cared and encouraged me, the Mdewakanton Sioux Community for chemical dependency treatment, and a host of others. Thank you.

I am forty-eight and this is a brief glimpse at the story of my life. I have raised two children. Have three grandchildren. Believe that God/Gitchi Manitou is my companion and helper in life's journey. I am single and a very independent woman who can stand on her own. I have reconciled with both of my parents. Genetic testing has since revealed that the man who raised me is really my biological father. However, I am grateful that I made the young choice to adopt Native Americans as my people and fathered my two children with a Native person. I have come to realize that every person has their own challenges and even demons to deal with. Every hurtful deed likely found its roots in that individual's own experience of abuse, neglect, addiction, or struggle. My present aspirations are to own the company I now work for, or, to move to Florida to live closer to my daughter and granddaughters.

You can take a bad/crappy life, turn it around, and have a good life. With help, I have done that. So can you.

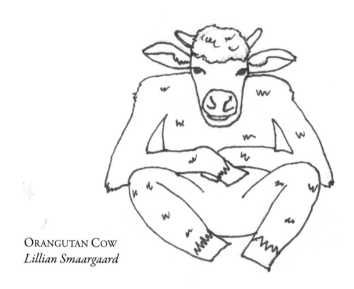

ORANGUTAN COW
Lillian Smaargaard

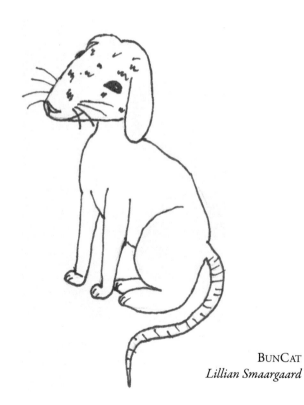

BUNCAT
Lillian Smaargaard

Tracy's Life

By Tracy Lyons

Some of these memories are very painful and it takes me a lot of thinking and fortitude to come forward with it. I was born October 28, 1952. By the time I was two months old I was deathly sick. Without the intervention of penicillin, most likely I would not be here today. This is the start of some of the heavy trauma that I've experienced in my life. Although, birth for the child and the mother is a very painful thing, also. Other than being sick a lot when I was really young, I would probably be an OK child. Until I reached about five years old when I started questioning who I was, I didn't seem to be like the rest of the girls.

In expressing this, I remember a lot of shame was brought on at that time and some corporal punishment. There were no girls in my neighborhood of my age, they were all boys. Somewhere after first grade in that summer, myself and three other neighborhood boys decided to dress up as women. My sister took some pictures of us. We had little hats with veils on them like some of the women wore of that time or before. At that time everything really clicked I understood that I was different. The next day, myself and the other three boys decided to play some house and I played the mother. We were at the three other boys houses. Their mother's name was Jeanette. She soon contacted my mother. Out of this I was brought more shame in doing that and some more corporal punishment.

As I type this out, tears are running down my cheek because I realized that this was a shameful thing and how parents can hurt their children so easily. At this time, I started not to reveal who I was and I started cross dressing when no one else was around. When I entered into 4th grade Halloween was coming up and I wanted to dress as a girl to be who I was. After long arguments with my mother, she finally gave in. At that time, I lived across the street from the Garfield school in northeast Brainerd. There is a house there now but it was just the field at that time. I would go home for lunch, then back to school. When home for lunch, I dressed as a girl in my older sister's blouse that was bright green large with green buttons on it. That's what I wore. I wore a skirt and a scarf when I went back to school. When I entered the school, it was just about time for classes to start and it was all OK at that time. And after school, we would line up on the West End of the school and my house was on the Far East end. Older boys grabbed me and groped me with teachers looking on. Nobody lifted a hand to help me. When I finally got home, my mother showed me no expression of sympathy. The neighborhood kids came over to pick me up to go trick-or-treating but I wouldn't go out. I finally went out by myself late in the evening walking alone. I realized that this time that I could not express myself that's who I was so, I went underground.

A long period of hiding soon followed when I still would cross dress when no one was around to express who I was. At Christmas time I would look in the Christmas catalog under all the things that the girls had to choose from for Christmas. I look at that little makeup things and dream but, it wasn't a dream that I could have.

I started going to church earlier in my life to a Baptist Church where I started learning verses and sin and God would send me to hell for sinning. As time goes on and as we mature as male born people, testosterone levels start to make me think that I was almost invisible. I started to drink early in life seemingly to hide who I was. You cannot escape with alcohol or drugs it's still there. I always had a hard time asking girls out for dates usually they asked me. I don't know if this was because of the way I am or because I am an introvert.

In high school, they had a tradition of Thursdays was queers day. This wasn't a positive thing this is searching for LGBT people to bash. Yes, I graduated from Brainerd high school in 1971 and this was a practice that went on. One learns to hide really well because you do not want to be attacked.

I finally met what was to be my wife and that's all I could put all this that I have spoken above behind me. I was also afraid that somebody may think of me as being gay. So, we got married really young but the struggle was still there. I started gathering my clothes and I kept them in a small briefcase with a lock on it in the bathroom of the apartment we lived in. Like a lot of newlyweds, a woman wants to explore what a man may hide so, when I got home from work I was questioned about it. I dressed in my clothes and there was a lot of shame placed on me at this time and she threatened to leave me. I got rid of all my clothes and I promised that I would never do this again.

Well, that was one promise that I could not keep I would continue to sneak around when no one was around cross dressing. This was continually on my mind torturing me over and over. I would do many male things – I would swing a 20 pound sledgehammer. I took up karate, and a lot of dangerous things. I drank a lot but could not escape. When I was in my 50s I was licensed to drive a big truck. At this time, they would send you through physical and urinalysis. My blood pressure started to rise. They put me on one blood pressure medicine but, it kept going up. The doctor put me on a second blood pressure medicine. They also cannot get my rapid pulse to slow down. I was heading for death because I was hiding from myself. The thoughts of suicide also came in at this time because I was sinning before God. I thought the only way I could escape hell was to commit suicide.

When I turned 61, I needed to see a therapist because I needed to start hormones to be myself. After a long time with the therapist, which is required before you can start estrogen which is a minimum of 12 weeks once a weeks, I received my first letter. On November 11, 2014, what is the first day then I took an antigen and was on estradiol patches. And out of this I no longer take any blood pressure medicine or rapid pulse medicine—I am who I am. My wife and I had argued many times and she moved out after driving four grandchildren that lived with us away. She said she wasn't a lesbian. We're still married at this time. This summer it'll be 51 years of marriage. She does come and see me on the weekends because I got tired and threatened her with divorce because I was too lonely. There's still many struggles in my life from very hurtful people. I had lost all my friends and it is very hard to build new ones especially being a trans woman.

I've had two surgeries since starting hormones breast augmentation and gender affirmation. I've lived full time since before 2014 who I am. In my life there have been many traumas besides the ones that I have mentioned with people trying to lay shame on me of who I am basically people who do not understand what goes on with the person which gender does not match their sex. I could tell you many more things but I'm over the parameters of the number of words that I was supposed to write.

Long Story Short

By Zannabella Gray Addison

I am Zannabella Lesla Gray! I was born in Crosby, Minnesota on August 1, 1988 to two young, unwed teenagers. There were a lot of struggles financially, especially after my parents had more children. We moved around quite a bit when I was little, including a big move to Iowa. My favorite things to do were rollerblade, ride my bike, read, and climb trees! When we moved back to Minnesota, I was in 5th grade. Everything was suddenly different. All of a sudden it MATTERED what I wore to school. There were trends that I could never keep up with, although I always tried.

When I got into the 7th grade things were even MORE different! I was going through a lot of hormonal changes and didn't fully comprehend what was going on. I also felt a lot of my parents' financial burden. They argued a lot and although they tried to fight "behind closed doors" there was still a lot of tension in the house. One memory I have about money is making a clock in wood shop and being afraid to ask for the $12 to bring it home. I knew money was a source of tension, so I didn't bother asking!

I had become obsessed with a boy in 8th grade, and we started dating that year, but he broke up with me over the summer. My best friend moved to a different school around that time too. So, on top of my hormones, I had catastrophic incidents in my life that really altered how I felt about myself. I was very depressed and attempted suicide. I didn't know how else to cope with the stress and changes I was dealing with. I began cutting my wrists and carving symbols into my skin. Self-mutilation was a way for me to release the pain I felt inside. It seems messed up, but my life was messed up.

At 13 years old I tried alcohol and weed for the first time. When I was 15, I started drinking to the point of intoxication. I was smoking cigarettes and weed regularly by age 16. 11th and 12th grade I was skipping school frequently to get high. A week before graduation, I tried meth. I spent the summer after high school doing every drug imaginable. I got pregnant that Fall and had my daughter in June 2007.

I want to back track a little and share the story about a train and fate. July

18th, 2006. I was huffing and driving. As I approached a railroad crossing, the lights started flashing and the arms went down. I thought that would be a perfect time to huff. I passed out and my car rolled into a moving train, totaling it out but leaving me without a scratch. A miracle! Afterwards I went to a friend's house, and I made a CD. I labeled it July 18th for the day that I hit the train. Over a year later, one of my friends found that CD and handed it to me. I realized then, that in my huffing stupor I had written JUNE 18th. Which is my daughter's birthday. On one of the worst days of my life, I was shown that I had a reason to live! THAT is more of a miracle than surviving the train!

I did end up cleaning up my act quite a bit and had two more children. Two boys a few years apart from each other. I was a server for many years and did my best to raise my kids on a low income. I had been in an abusive relationship and eventually chose to be a single mom. One of the biggest barriers for me was finding childcare. Life was tough, but in 2017 it became even harder. I had started doing drugs again, shortly after my 29th birthday and my world was ripped apart within a few short months. I had been in and out of emergency rooms, the grace unit and psych wards due to drug-induced psychosis. It was the absolute worst part of my life. I ended up with another abusive boyfriend and lost custody of my children. Thankfully, all three of them were placed with their grandparents. Losing my kids tore a hole in my heart.

I finally got clean in 2019 and started the amazing journey of recovery! I have been clean off meth for over 4 years now and have experienced so many blessings along the way! My fiancé, Tyler, and I met when I was a little over a year clean and he was a few months sober. We have my two older kids over a couple times a month, plus he has a daughter from a previous relationship, so I have a bonus child! I pray every day for my little guy that lives with a different set of grandparents. I haven't seen him since he was 2 and he's almost 8-years-old! I know that he is in good hands though and that helps ease my mind. My soul calls out to him often.

Tyler and I had a baby boy last year on my 3-year anniversary of being clean. Our little guy is such a blessing! His birth was a sign that I am where I need to be. I have made mistakes, yes, but I try to be the best version of myself that I can be. Tyler and I are getting married on August 31st and we are looking forward to spending the rest of our life together! He is an insurance agent for National Insurance Brokers and a recovery coach for MN Adult and Teen Challenge. I currently work for Lakes Area Restorative Justice. I am also in the process of publishing my first book!

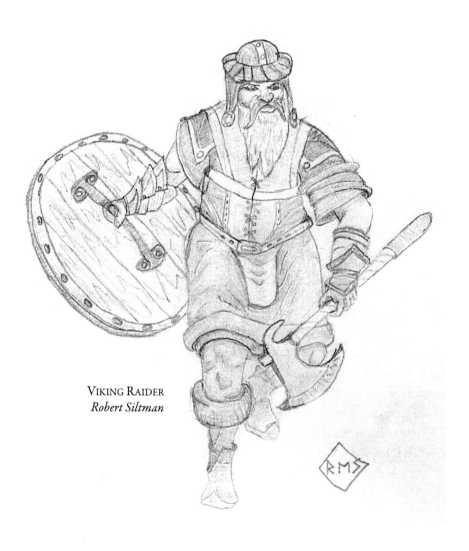

VIKING RAIDER
Robert Siltman

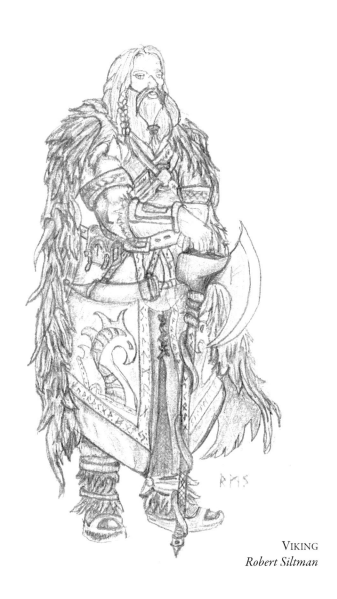

VIKING
Robert Siltman

Breaking the Cycle

Anonymous

Lexi entered the small room, put her three-month-old daughter, Aiyana, in her car seat for a nap and sat down at the round table. Pausing to contemplate where to begin, it seemed that chronological order would best reveal the cycles in her life and her present desire to break them.

Lexi was born in Colombia, a member of the Huila people, and was adopted by a couple in Minneapolis when she was just a baby. She was raised there, the second adopted child of her adoptive parents.

"It was hard to grow up not having anyone of the same color in my family," Lexi began. "All the kids in schools were white. My parents enrolled me in a private Catholic school, which added to the strangeness. I never connected to the faith. It just increased my disconnect."

So upsetting was the disconnect that her parents removed her from private school and enrolled her in public school. Still, 98% of the kids were white, and Lexi struggled to fit in. She began therapy at the age of 11. Her anger was later identified as part of "adoption/abandonment" issues often felt by adoptees and intensified in kids who are adopted internationally.

"My parents followed the advice of their therapist," Lexi explained, "and put me into an out-patient program at Prairie St. John's. They did the best they could with the tools they were given, but I was nearly at a black-out state. During my pre-teen and teen years, I felt the world was against me."

These memories are returning as Lexi's own 11-year-old daughter is experiencing a disconnect in her life. Lexi is working through transgenerational trauma, recognizing the past in her daughter's present. By age 15, Lexi's treatments included Adderall, Ritalin, Ambien – a menu of amphetamines prescribed to her repeatedly throughout her youth. The response to her struggles? More drugs. Now, Lexi is making choices to stop the cycle.

"I did find sanctuary in sports, at that time. I was naturally a good athlete. I was on the high school varsity team even as a middle-schooler. I excelled but,"

Lexi continued, "I realized by age 16 that the Adderall affected me. It increased my heart rate, producing anxiety. Once, on the field, I had an asthma attack and that ended my sports."

Oxycodone was added to her list of drugs when, also at age 16, she had her gallbladder removed. It "hooked" her. During this time, she lost her best friend to drugs. Soon after this death, she moved to Red Lake, where she met the father of her oldest two children. Dan was heavily into opiates and was an alcoholic. He already had two children.

"Dan was sober for most of the years we were together," Lexi related. "I became the mom to his kids and we had two of our own. Then, Dan relapsed in 2016. He got crazy, mean, scary crazy. He tried to kill me, and unfortunately, my daughter, four-years-old at the time, witnessed it. I felt stuck there, believing I had to stay for the kids, but now we had to get out. I felt the horror that I saw in my daughter's eyes. This had to stop. Dan's kids chose to go with me. That made me a single mom with four kids!" Lexi's parents had received a call from a neighbor, suspecting her abuse. Her parents drove up that day to retrieve her and the kids. She and the kids lived with her parents in Minneapolis while she got back on her feet.

2016 was a pivotal year for Lexi in multiple ways. It was also the year she found out her birth mother, Graciella, was alive, still living in Colombia, and had children. Lexi recalls the pain of discovering that Graciella had, and kept, three of her children. "I remember calling my mom after I found my birthmother on Facebook. I sent my mom screenshots and practically screamed, 'Is it her? Is it her? She has kids, Mom; how could she do that!' The pain stabbed. My mom confirmed it was Graciella and reminded me that we did not yet know her story. Together, we worked on messages to reach out to her."

A year later, Lexi and Graciella met. When Lexi and her mom searched the Bogota airport for her, they spotted a large group of people with balloons and posters; they were smiling and waving excitedly. "When I saw my birthmother, something clicked. I look like her; we hold our bodies the same, our hands, our shoulders; we walk the same. Everyone commented. While my anger faded, questions arose. We shared our stories on Graciella's balcony that night. Everyone was crying. The doctors at the orphanage told her I had died as a baby, and the orphanage told us, when we visited for my 12th birthday, that Graciella had died. The pack of lies that came out hurt and bonded us at the same time. Forgiveness is healing. I believe that experiences like mine were what the Creator intended to bring all people in the world together."

Lexi brought with her to Colombia the Adderall, Xanax, and Benzodiazepine medications from her childhood. "The different doctors didn't even know, or check, what the others were doing. I now realize the mix could've been deadly," Lexi recalled. While in Colombia, a birth uncle noticed all the medications she was taking and asked her, why, what were they for?

"My uncle was visiting from Australia," Lexi recounted. "He knew English and became the translator for us. One day, he faced me with, 'When you want to change your life, let me know.'" And one day, Lexi was ready. She went with him on a nine-hour drive into the mountains of Colombia. "We did ceremonies. I sat out for two nights and three days. He shared the story of his past addiction to alcohol. I finally faced mine to drugs. I came off EVERYTHING! I was detoxed from everything, and I had made an important connection that remains intact today. He is one of my biggest supporters."

During one of the ceremonies, it was revealed to Lexi that she was a "plant" worker. That her life-calling involved natural (plant) medicines and wholistic healing. This revelation manifested itself into a passion and her future work in Brainerd.

Once back, Lexi became aware of Valhalla Place, a medical clinic with addiction counselling and methadone programs. "You can just walk in and sign up as a patient. You can get medications for withdrawal and opioid disorders." Nine months later, Lexi was ready to take the next step.

In 2018, Four Winds Lodge Program entered the picture with a new element: Culture. Beyond behavior, trauma, and drug counseling, it offered Native American culture. "The healing came from an Indigenous base. We did sweat lodges and ritualistic ceremonies," Lexi related. "That was cool! That was something my parents knew nothing about when they sent me to therapy." She graduated from Four Winds and, in 2020, returned to help others.

Lexi worked as a cultural assistant at Four Winds briefly, giving her the opportunity to use plants. With plant donations from Central Lakes College greenhouse, Lexi incorporated growing foods, healthy diets, and the concepts of natural healing into the program's emphasis.

Lexi credits Central Lakes College's META-5 program for displaced homemakers and TRIO, a support program guiding students to graduation, as major factors in her recovery journey. "In order to break the cycle of mental illness and addiction, one has to have a network—a community," Lexi insisted. "It is not easy to reach out and find support when you are at a low point. I credit Kimberly Pilgrim, the head of META-5, with saving my life."

META-5 provides assertiveness training, support groups and retreats. "The women's gatherings got me out of my everyday life. Connections with other women through retreats were pivotal in my recovery. We went to Duluth, Grand Marais, places outside of Brainerd. It filled us. These times were a beautiful thing!"

"Otherwise, I've been alone since I left Dan. Then, in 2020, Dan, the father of our children, had a mental health crisis. He attempted suicide. I was taking finals at college when I received the call to get myself and the kids to the hospital to say good-bye. Although I was healthy at the time, after seeing Dan, I realized more than ever that I could not afford to screw up anymore. The reality of life or death stared me in the face. My kids were counting on me. In addition, a man who abused and tried to kill me was a big part of my adult experience. I looked at the man who 'survived' with for six years with our children and knew I was done; I had to be done. It was time to bury that old life for myself and my kids so we could move forward.

"Miraculously, Dan survived, but he was changed. He remembered his kids, but seemed far away, not present. The kids are dealing with that. We all need support systems.

"Support systems can be hard to find, but they are here in Brainerd if you look. Find your community and be involved. I'm working with ceremonies, Recovery gardens, Up Front and the 12-step program. As Indigenous people, we're supposed to give, then life gives back. Incredibly, in 2022, we were chosen for a Habitat for Humanity house. I'll be able to put down roots and raise my kids here. I was giving and that is when HFH gave back.

"It's about breaking the cycle," she said, looking down at Aiyana, asleep at her feet. "After living with us for a short time, Aiyana's dad relapsed into a mental health crisis. I had to make him leave—for the kids and for me. No more. Breaking the cycle is not easy, but it must be done.

"I'm grateful to the good people I've found in Brainerd. Being part of a community helps," Lexi added. "Brainerd could do a lot more to support the Indigenous culture. Currently, it has a statue—that of Babe the Waabigwan Ox downtown, painted by Aiyana Beaulieu; we can do better," Lexi smiled.

"People need a supportive network to help them navigate and connect," she concludes. "You give what you can, and you will get back."

Lexi picked up Aiyana. "You have to break the cycle. You do it for yourself and for your kids."

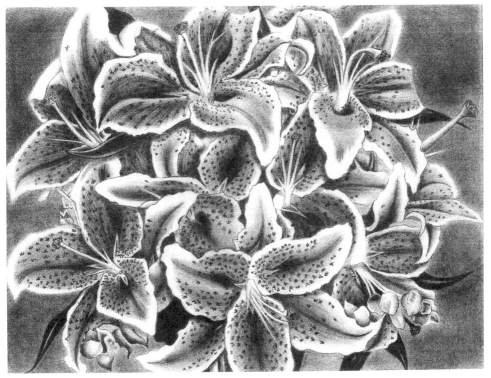

TIGER LILIES
Jason Lowry

Michael Erickson

By Michael Erickson

I am a transracially adopted Japanese American, 67 year old male, who has lived most of my life in Minnesota. I was born in Tokyo and adopted there by white parents who had no idea what it meant to raise a child of a different color. I remember my first day of kindergarten. I was greeted with, "Hey Jap, where's your bayonet?" My school experiences tended to go downhill from there as well as many experiences outside of school. There were many fights caused by racial slurs and insults over the years. My father taught me how to fight. My mother told me Jesus loves all the little children of the world—red, yellow, black, and white. I hated that song. I did not feel loved by Jesus or the world.

I was 5 when I stood in a St Paul court room with many other non-citizens to take an oath that meant I would become a United States citizen. I vividly remember going home and looking in the mirror fully expecting to somehow look blonde with round blue eyes. I was so deeply disappointed that I still looked like the old me. How stupid could I have been to think things would have been different.

Transracial adoption manufactures creatures of marginality. The outside world perceives you as one thing and yet you are entirely different on the inside. For example, as a Japanese adopted by white parents I grew up internalizing pretty much everything white, but the outside world perceived my yellow skin and saw me as a Jap, Chink, slant eyes, someone who can't say their Rs, etc. In other words a Banana, yellow on the outside and white on the inside.

Children of color who are raised in primarily white families grow up with mixed racial identities. I was a Banana. Apples are red on the outside, but white on the inside. While others are Oreos, black on the outside and white on the inside. All these terms deny one's authentic personhood. You truly never really belong anywhere. You have no tribe.

Years later, while doing graduate school studies I was working with families who had transracially adopted Korean children. I was unique to them as I was an adult who had lived through the experience. I could share this with the children and the parents. The one constant question the parents always asked was, 'Do you think it will be easier now for my child than it was for you?" My answer was always, no. I still do not see significant progress in race relations in our community or nation.

Racism and prejudices are everywhere. They haven't gone away. They may have become more refined, went underground, or just become more in your face bigoted. None the less they are alive and well.

The reality that I see is that it is now more dangerous than ever to be non-white. Hate groups and White Supremacists, according to the FBI, are our country's number one internal threat. Within the last year, hate crimes against Asian Americans went up 300%.

I would like to lIve in a world where there was no hatred, no war, no hunger, no strife, and each person was judged by the merit of the worthiness of their being and not by the color of their skin, their religion, or their gender. That would be great, but it seems we have difficulty achieving that in our own country or state. Martin Luther King Jr stated, "Injustice anywhere is a threat to justice everywhere."

Over time I've never found my tribe. At some point, I would like to live in a Minnesota where when someone asks "Where are you from" and I reply that I am from Baxter, Minnesota they do not come back with "But where are you really from?" At that point perhaps the tears from my hurt will start to put the fire of my anger out.

Beauty With-in

By Michael LaFlex

Why couldn't they look at me before like that?
They just saw me as an ugly bug.
My beauty was within, just waiting for the right
moment to show.
It was always there, but all they saw was an ugly
bug.
All they needed to do was have patience and let
me show my beauty when I was ready.
It was always there.
They just chose not to see it.

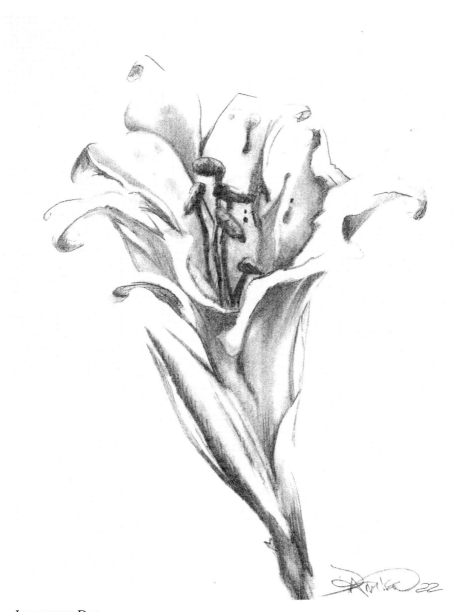

LILY OF THE DAY
Damien Graham

Imagine This

By Patricia Adell Dickson

ist definition: a follower of a distinctive practice

Take the ist* away
From social distancing and
Dancing is what's left.

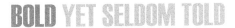

Floaty Place Fetty Ways

By Jeremy Cadwell

Big addicted to Fetty
Neva leave the Fetty
I love the way the Fetty melts away
Love the way it takes me away
To a lovely floaty place
Need to change my ways
But Fetty always screaming my name
I need to change lanes
Fetty takes away the pain
There's nothing that will change the Fetty ways
Always chasing a bag stocking mule
Until I fall back to the Fetty bag
Man, Fetty is a dark place
Always worried about Fetty
That lovely floaty place
I strayed away from my family
'Cause Fetty takes me to a lovely floaty place
Lovely floaty days

FOOTNOTE—Fetty is a slang term for fentanyl. The author wrote this poem while a resident of the Crow Wing County Jail. When he was released he went to a homeless shelter and died of an overdose one week later.

Jessicorn

By Jessica Stewart

I am more than black and white
I am every shade of gray
I'll try to paint a picture
with my words on this page

I'm a complex contradiction
made of contours, depth and breadth
A bipolar roller coaster
You never know what's next

I walk the borderline between I hate you and don't leave me
General anxiety holds me back and leads me
down the rocky, winding path
from dysthymia to manic

I exist on my own planet
where I want you all to live
I want you all to love me,
though I have nothing to give

I don't care what you think about me
Someone please accept me
I don't need your acceptance
Please don't reject me

I'm paradoxical
I'm paralaxical

I wax poetic in ways you'll never know
I'm a unicorn in a human uniform
At the end of the day
there's no one quite like me

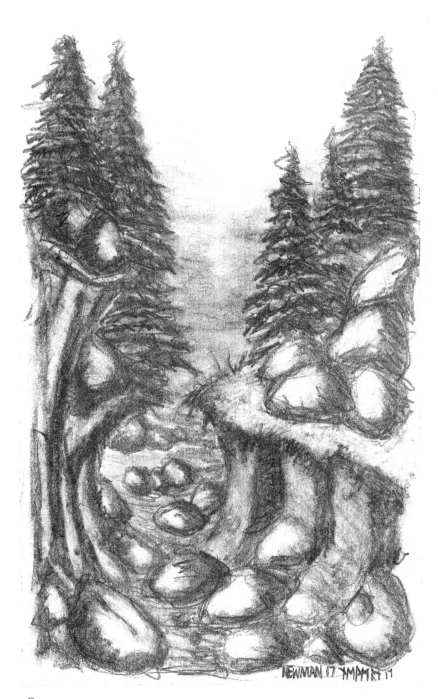

CREVASS
Ken Newman

Afterword

It is my privilege to be asked to contribute to this story project and share some community wide resources to you the reader. In Crow Wing County, we are privileged to have the community health movement: **Crow Wing Energized (CWE)**. It is lead by Essentia Health and Crow Wing County and receives money from the Statewide Health Improvement Partnership. Our Mission: A grassroots movement to improve health and wellness in our community making the healthy choice the easy choice. We focus on our physical health and our mental health. Why? Because, we know that nationally, 1 in 5 people live with a mental illness; in Crow Wing County, 1 in 4 people live with a mental illness. Through our **Mental Fitness Goal Group and Adverse Childhood Experiences (ACEs)** and **Resiliency Coalition (ARC)**, we have continued to work on our overall mental well-being, stigma reduction, and suicide prevention. Since we have hosted training to become a Make It OK ambassador or an ACE facilitator trainer, we have volunteers that will come to your place of work, place of worship, and/or community event or gathering; there is NO cost. Listed below are some mental health resources in our area; this list is not all-inclusive by any means.

- **988: Help is available.** IF you need help, dial **988**.

- **NAMI: National Alliance on Mental Illness:**
  www.nami.org

- **SAMHSA: Substance Abuse and Mental Health Services Administration:** www.samhsa.gov/find-help/national-helpline
  o **SAMHSA** National Helpline: 1-800-662-4357

- **Make It OK**
  www.makeitok.org

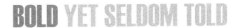
BOLD YET SELDOM TOLD

- **Bridges of Hope**
  www.bridgesofhopemn.org
    o **Warming Shelter**: overnight shelter
    www.bridgesofhopemn.org/warmingshelter

- **Central Minnesota Adult & Teen Challenge**: 218-833-8777
  Brainerd Addiction Treatment & Recovery Center
  www.mntc.org/Brainerd

- **12 Step Programs**
    o **Upfront Alano Society of Brainerd**: 302 Fourth Ave NE;
    Brainerd, MN 56401 – 218-828-4811
    o **Lakes Area Alano Association**; 7829 Minnesota Hwy 210;
    Baxter, MN 56425 – 218-825-3770

- **The Shop**:723 Washington Street; Brainerd, Mn 56401 218-454-0009

- **Crow Wing County Community Services**; 204 Laurel Street, #31;
  Brainerd, MN 56401 218-824-1140

- **Essentia Health – Substance Use**
  www.essentiahealth.org/services/substance-use-disorder

- **Crow Wing Energized**: www.crowwingenergized.org

- **Resourceful** – free community resource guide
  www.weareresourceful.org

- **Food Resources**: See **Crow Wing Energized** and **Resourceful**

I am grateful for our community members who were brave enough and willing to share their stories; you are the reason I continue to be passionate about the work we do as well as give me hope for our future.

Submitted by Karen Johnson, Crow Wing Energized, Community Health Specialist

Acknowledgements

In addition to the writers and artists who contributed to book, there were many others who worked behind the scenes to make this project happen. They served various roles such as fund raising, editing, publishing, marketing, ghost writing, and general organizing of the project. These valuable people include:

Wendy Adamson
Brian Andrews
Lilia Behr
Chip Borkenhagen
Jean Borkenhagen
Jennifer DeVries
Christine Grossman
Dan Hegstad
Jeff Howard
Karen Johnson
Lowell Johnson
Janet Kurtz
Miranda Neuwirth
Maurice Olson
Darrell Pederson
TyAnne Rezac
Donna Sallie
Ann Schwartz
Krista Soukup

A huge thank you for your support of the Crow Wing Community Stories Project!

Reader's Guide

Readers and writers have a unique connection. Artists and art appreciators also do. Let's call the people who are featured in this book 'creators', who all are engaging in creative expression through art and writing. The featured creators in *Bold Yet Seldom Told* don't know who will choose to read the book. You, the reader, holding this copy in your hands, will engage with them when you empathize with the characters and images, and relate to their situations in your own unique way. Maybe you will be challenged when you use your imagination to visualize and understand the perspective? Even though we may not have had the same experiences as the writers and artists are sharing, we all still construct meaning from their work.

This 'meaning making' is what reading teachers call comprehension. But when you add 'ion' to the end of a word it shows the act or result of doing something. This implies the end. You did something. It's over. You went to the gallery and gazed at the sculptor. You finished the last chapter. You will process the stories and images using your background or worldview (what reading teachers call 'schema'). And, just like a great movie you saw the night before and woke up still thinking about, you may continue to reflect and relate to the image, the story. This thinking is an ongoing action. Comprehending. The 'ing' versus the 'ion' implies that you are questioning, reflecting, learning, and growing. It's fostering a sense of connection and shared experience around the stories and images that stick with us. Connection is the energy that exists between people when they feel seen, heard, and valued. The relationship between the artist and art appreciator, or the reader and the writer, cannot be understated. It's deeply personal.

To move further along in the comprehending and meaning making process, you may ask others who have read the book some questions. You might ask, "What do you think the author meant when they wrote 'then his Shawshank Redemption moment came?'" If you haven't seen that movie, talking with someone who has will enhance understanding what that phrase might mean. And together you can examine and discuss what emotions or concepts are intended to be communicated. Is the painting or drawing more about exploration of ideas? Or is there an agenda she or he is promoting? If so, what might that agenda be?

When we were kids, teachers were really into asking basic questions about the stories we would read. For example, "What year did Chris's father die?" Is this a question that will lead to a rich discussion? Or is this a question that might simply 'prove' that I read the book? Ask instead, "Alvin wrote that his first experience of feeling different was when his 2nd grade teacher made him wear a brace so his shaky handwriting could be improved. Have you ever been made to feel different by someone in a position of authority?" That's a text to self connection. Or you might think, "That story reminds me of another story I read. In that story...". That is a text to text connection. You can also make a text to world connection, where you think "The situation in this story reminds me of something I heard about happening in...".

We are confident that if you participate in meaningful discussions about the art and stories in *Bold Yet Seldom Told*, you will build connections with the creators, with others who are reading this book, and hopefully you will also strengthen the connections in your own mind that lead you towards a deeper understanding of how we are all, well, connected.

Questions to Guide Discussion

We hope that the following questions may help encourage diverse opinions and interpretations for a lively discussion. These questions are meant to be a springboard for exploring deeper themes, symbolism, and intentions. You might consider sharing these questions ahead of time, so that discussion participants have time to reflect on the book and prepare their thoughts. Select a facilitator who can pose the questions and encourage universal participation and active listening, and expect the book discussion to foster a sense of community around the book's stories and images.

What overarching themes do you see recurring throughout these stories?

How did the mood or tone of each story or artwork affect your emotional engagement?

Are there any connections or common threads between different stories in the collection?

Did any stories offer insights into cultural or societal issues? Which ones and how?

Did any story resonate with personal experiences or beliefs you hold? Share your reflections.

How did the stories affect your perspective on certain topics or emotions?

Sincerely,

Lowell Johnson & TyAnne Guida Rezac